WORLD RECORD WEBER

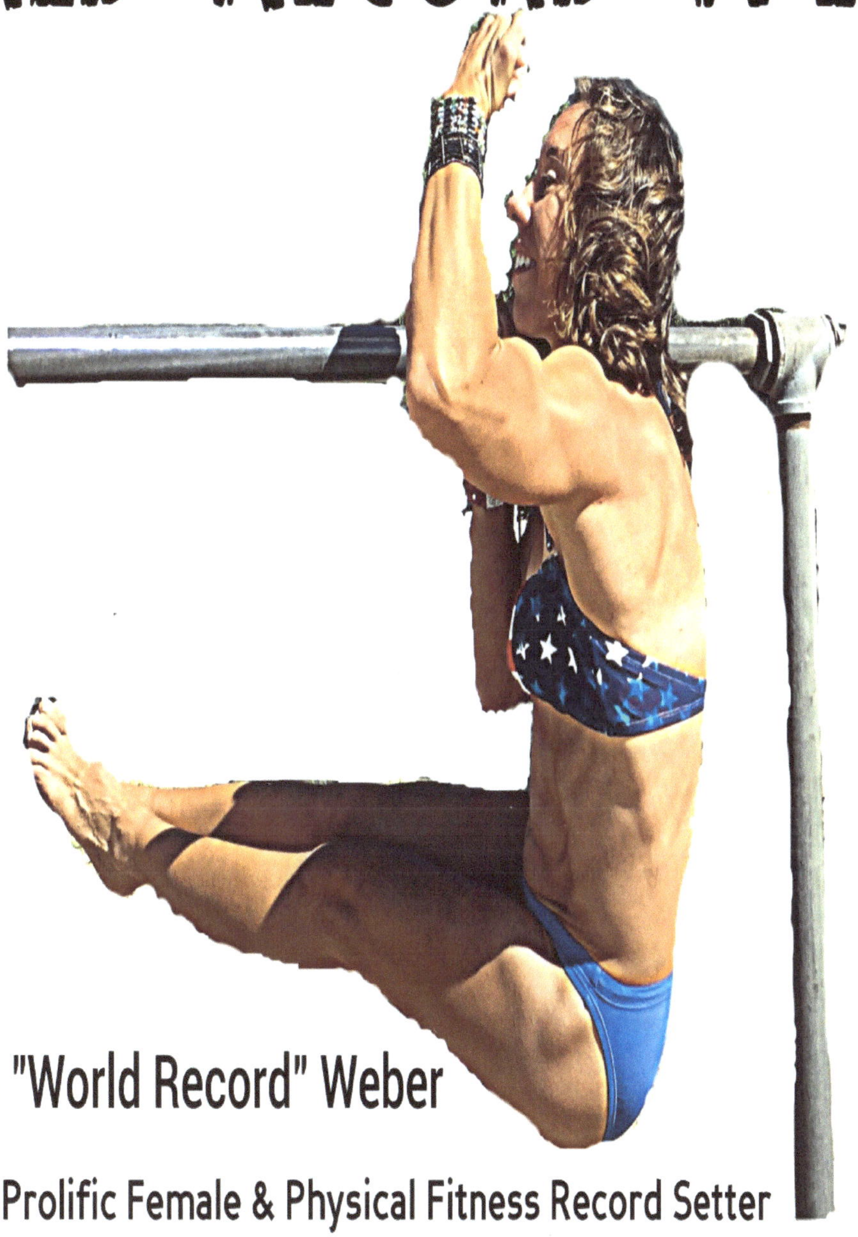

By: Alicia "World Record" Weber

World's Most Prolific Female & Physical Fitness Record Setter

WELLNESS ROUTINES

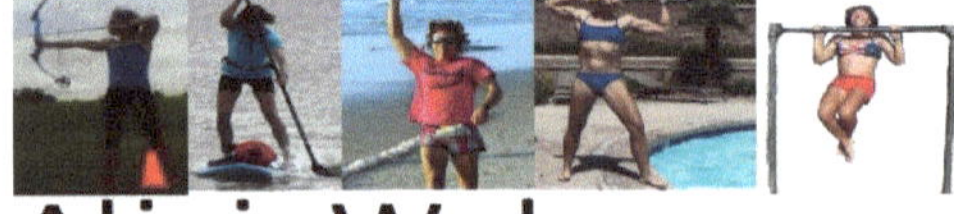

Introduction to Alicia "World Record" Weber

Alicia Weber is known as the Barrier Breaker Coach where she guides people with medical conditions and various obstacles and turns them into Champions in Sports and Life. She is a degreed fitness and wellness professional (20+ years), published author of 3 books, and founder of The Weber Way to Wellness (AliciaWeber.com).

Alicia has been competing as an elite athlete for 26 years (as of 2018). She represented the USA in 7 World Championships and she won National, North American, and World Championship titles. She also holds more than 500 world records in physical fitness events (first overall out of men and women). According to Recordsetter World Records (world's most popular record book), Alicia has been the World's Most Prolific Female Record Setter, since 2012. Alicia is about teaching effective, innovative wellness methods where people can see results quickly, while having a lot of fun in the process.

Educational Background

Alicia competed as a student-athlete at the University of Florida where she received her Bachelor 's degree in Telecommunication and Film Studies in 2002. She ran under the Olympic Coach, JJ Clark. She became the first UF letter-winning track and cross country runner to turn pro in triathlon from 2004-2008. A prominent UF speaker and entertainer, Alicia received a special award for her inspirational motivational speaking, while on the Gator cross country team in 2000.

After UF, Alicia continued her pursuit for excellence as a self-coached athlete as she continued to work on more degrees till age 31. She earned a Bachelor's degree in Biology and then spent two years in a Doctorate of Physical Therapy Program. She left the program when she realized she did not want to be a DPT, but she wanted to focus on medical massage therapy. Alicia transferred into a massage therapy program and received her license with specialties in medical and sport massage in 2011.

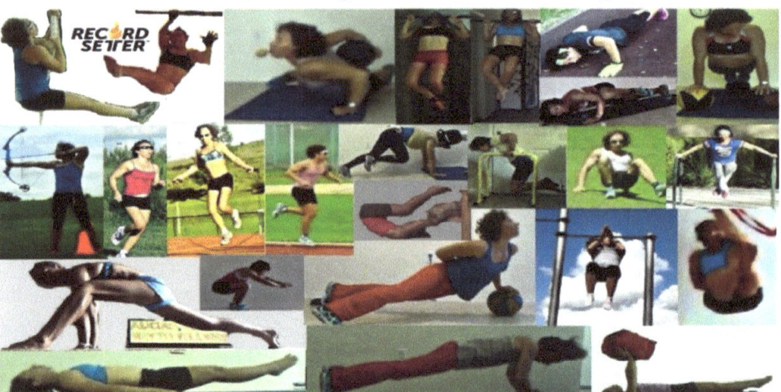

Athletic Career Highlights and Results

The two accomplishments Alicia is most proud of so far are the following: Becoming the first human to officially set 1,000 physical fitness world records covering all five areas of fitness and Becoming the Most Decorated 10K Beach Runner in the history of the sport (winning 3 titles, setting 2 course records, taking second place 3 times, and third place once...over 7 years).

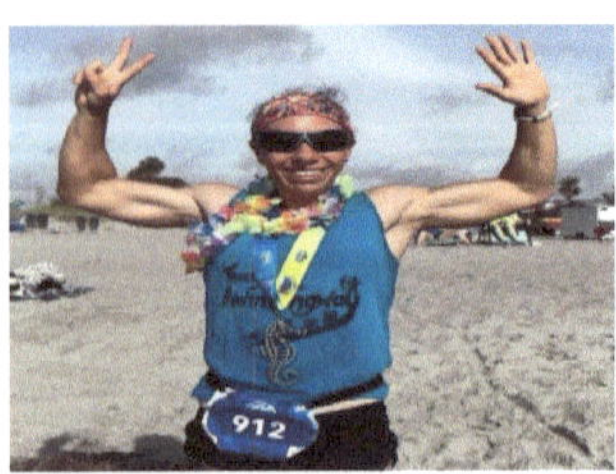

Alicia has completed a long series of studies on herself and clients ages 3-97 over the course of 9 years (2009-2018). She discovered wellness routines that promote building bone density, prevent injuries, and enhance athletic performance. She reveals these secret wellness routines in this book to help you become your best. She adds "WRW Facts" that relate to the wellness routines to demonstrate how they help with producing her success. Note: WRW stands for World Record Weber.

World Record Weber Wellness Routines

Written By Alicia "World Record" Weber

ISBN 0-9722754-2-8

Copyright © 2018 Alicia Weber

This book is NOT intended to treat an illness or disease or help a person that is under care of a physician, or following a special diet and exercise program to treat an illness or disease.

The author gives general guidelines, proven methods, and instructions, but <u>not a personalized program.</u> The author is not responsible (as a matter of product liability, negligence, or otherwise) for any injury resulting from the material in this book.

Table of Contents

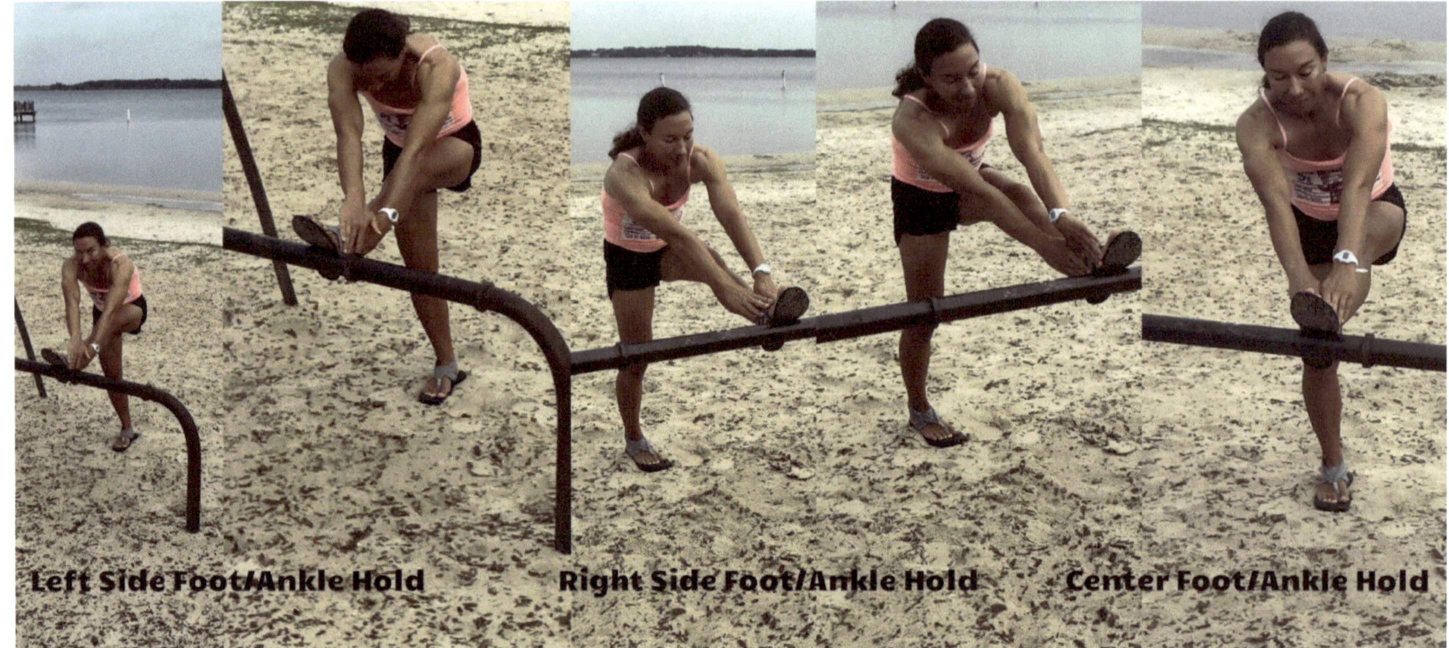

3 Location Hamstring Stretch (3 x 30 second Holds)

Purpose: World Record Weber considers this stretch the absolute most important stretch you can do before ANY exercise. She has been doing this stretch everyday, since Elementary School to prevent hamstring injuries and develop hamstring flexibility.

Goal: Keep both legs straight and forward. The foot of standing leg when pointed forward helps to stretch Abdominals and Hip Flexors. Touch the sides of your foot on the side holds. Touch your toes or front of your foot on center holds.

Progressions: Work to holding a straight, stretched out leg at least to waist level. Some people may need to start by using a one foot or two foot table or stool. Only one 30 second hold per position is necessary. Extra sets can be done though.

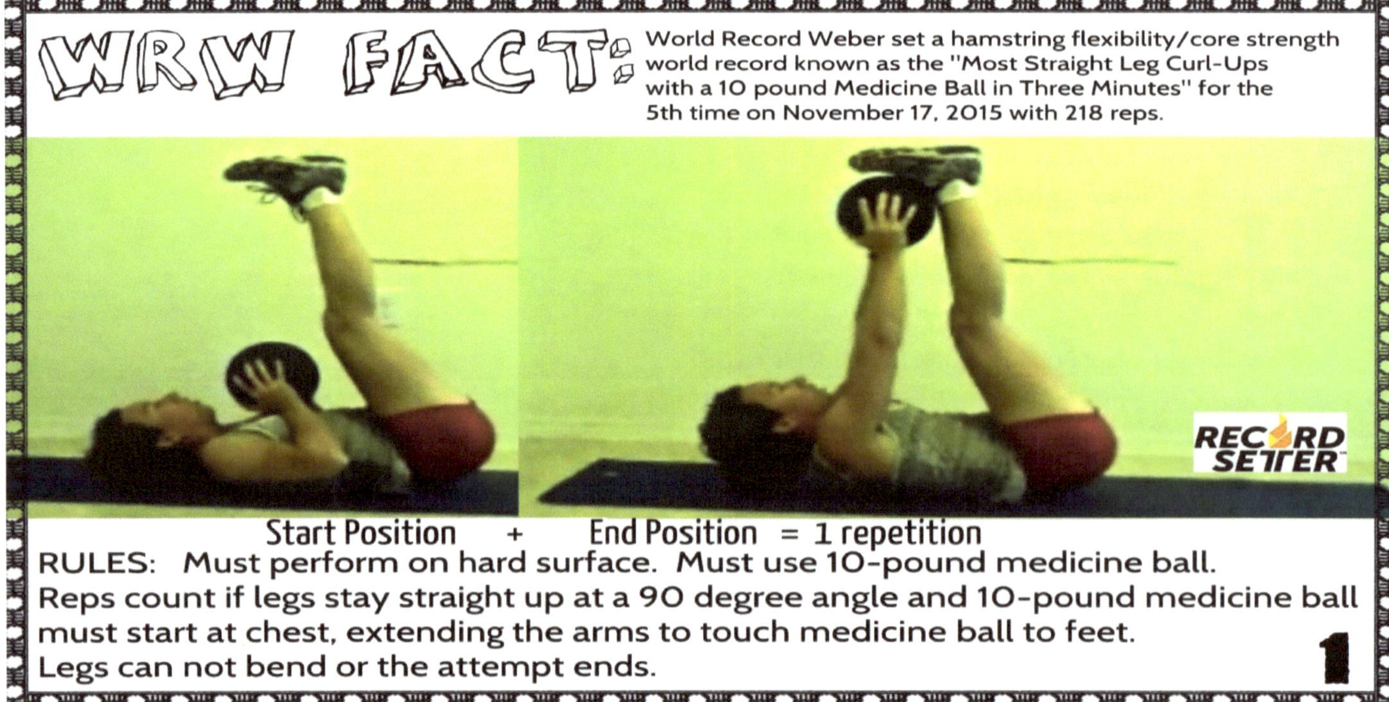

RULES: Must perform on hard surface. Must use 10-pound medicine ball. Reps count if legs stay straight up at a 90 degree angle and 10-pound medicine ball must start at chest, extending the arms to touch medicine ball to feet. Legs can not bend or the attempt ends.

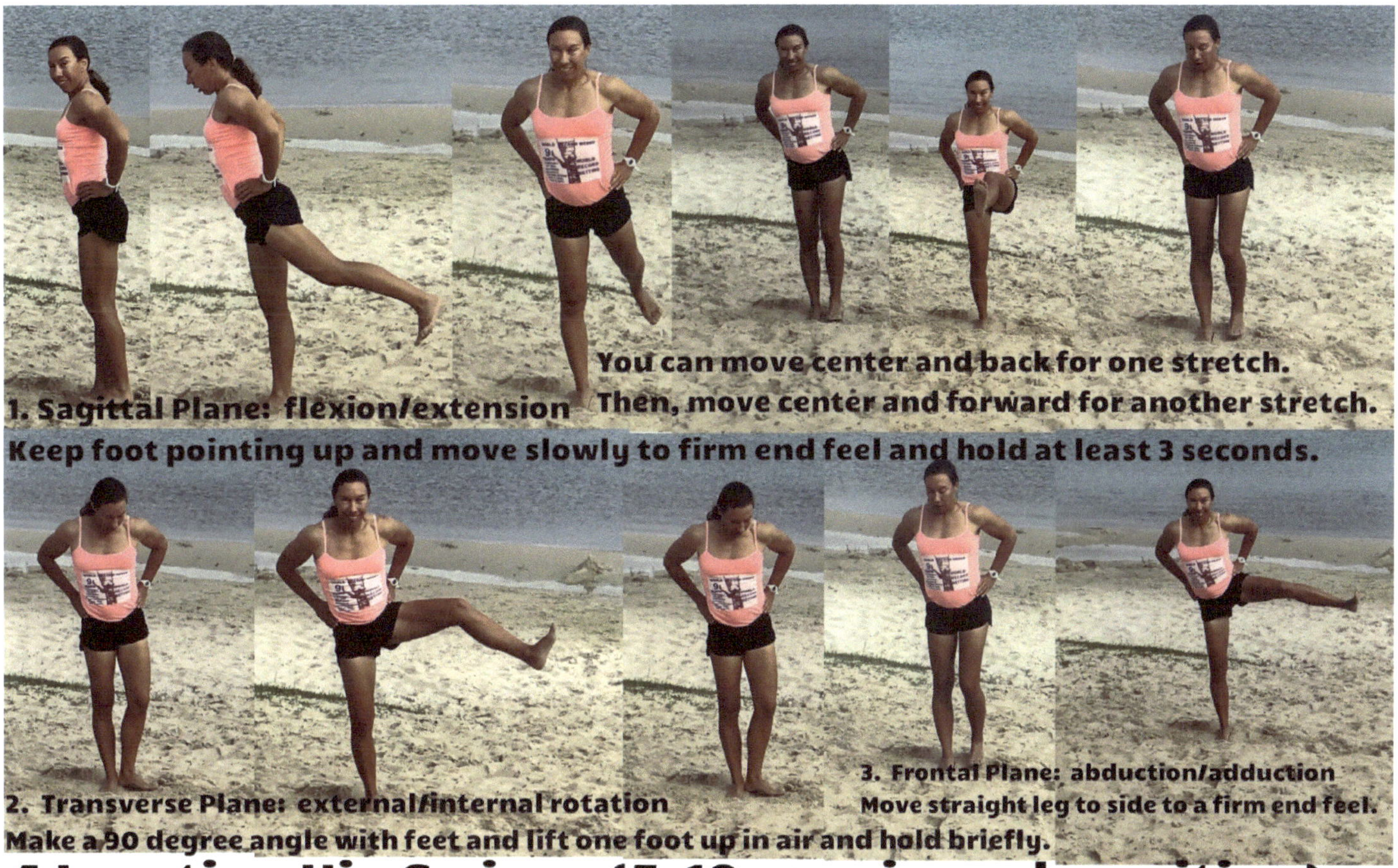

1. Sagittal Plane: flexion/extension
You can move center and back for one stretch.
Then, move center and forward for another stretch.
Keep foot pointing up and move slowly to firm end feel and hold at least 3 seconds.
2. Transverse Plane: external/internal rotation
Make a 90 degree angle with feet and lift one foot up in air and hold briefly.
3. Frontal Plane: abduction/adduction
Move straight leg to side to a firm end feel.

4 Location Hip Swings (5-10 reps in each position)

Goal: We will work all three angles of the hip joint as we smoothly transition into each movement, while balancing on one foot. Repeat on both sides. This stretch builds healthy balance, ROM, and flexibility.

WRW FACT:

On February 23, 2015 Alicia set the World Record for the "Fastest One-Leg 500 Meter Row (Rower Under 136 lbs.)" when she clocked 2:06.80 only using her left leg.

In 2016 Alicia became one of just a few lightweight female indoor rowers in the 33 year history of the Southern Sprints World Qualifier to win double gold in the 500 meter & 2,000 meter.

RECORD SETTER

One Leg Rowing recruits single extremity strength and activates muscle stabilizers.

One Leg Rowing recruits single extremity strength and activates muscle stabilizers.

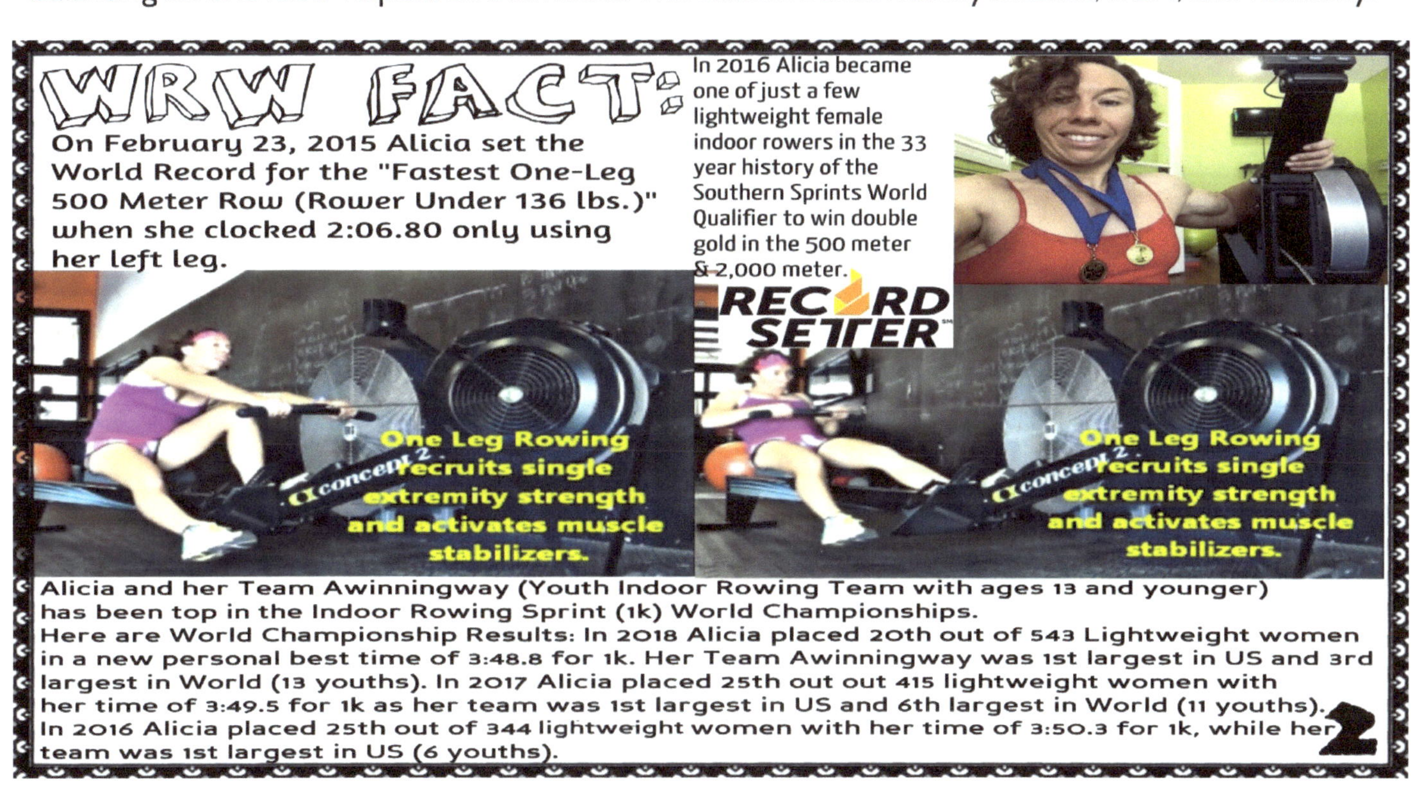

Alicia and her Team Awinningway (Youth Indoor Rowing Team with ages 13 and younger) has been top in the Indoor Rowing Sprint (1k) World Championships.
Here are World Championship Results: In 2018 Alicia placed 20th out of 543 Lightweight women in a new personal best time of 3:48.8 for 1k. Her Team Awinningway was 1st largest in US and 3rd largest in World (13 youths). In 2017 Alicia placed 25th out out 415 lightweight women with her time of 3:49.5 for 1k as her team was 1st largest in US and 6th largest in World (11 youths). In 2016 Alicia placed 25th out of 344 lightweight women with her time of 3:50.3 for 1k, while her team was 1st largest in US (6 youths).

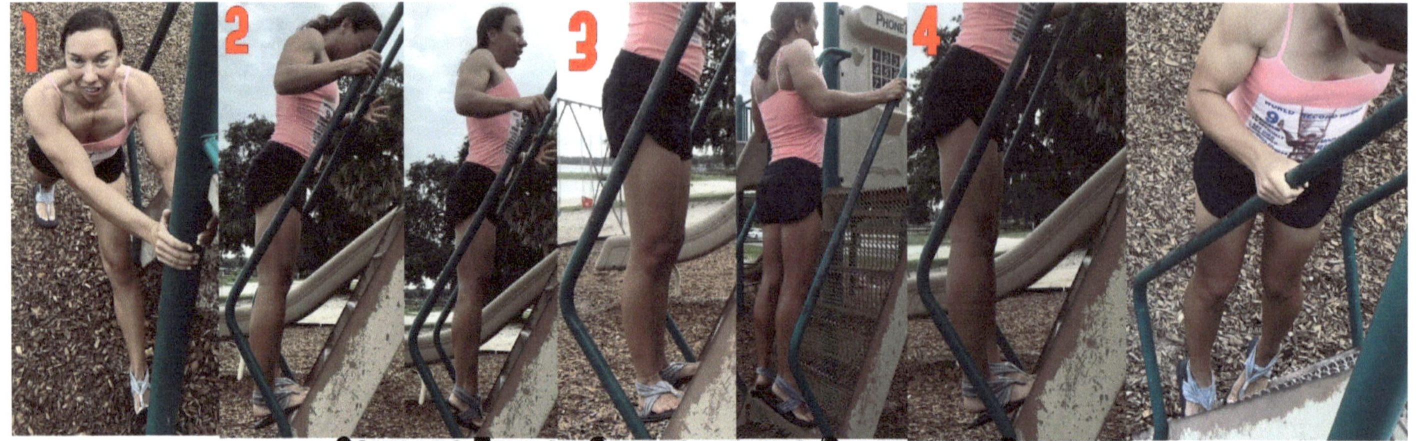

Achilles Tendon Strengthening/Stretching Routine

(Follow in order of pictures. Begin with Achilles stretch followed by one set of 5-10 reps of each type of toe raise.)

Purpose: Perform routine before any fast moving sports training i.e. sprinting, basketball, volleyball, and soccer. This routine has been shown to prevent and heal achilles tendonitis. It strengthens and stretches achilles tendon and calf muscle to prevent injuries.

Goal: Toe raises are slow and controlled working full ROM. Best performed on a step as shown to maximize stretch. Follow order of pictures: 1. 30 Second Achilles Tendon stretch (both legs), 2. Feet Together Toe Raises, 3. Heels Together Toe Raises, 4. Toes Toward Each Other Toe Raises, 5. One Leg Forward One Leg Toe Raises, 6. One Leg Everted (foot pointing out) Toe Raises, and 7. One Leg Inverted (foot pointing in) Toe Raises.

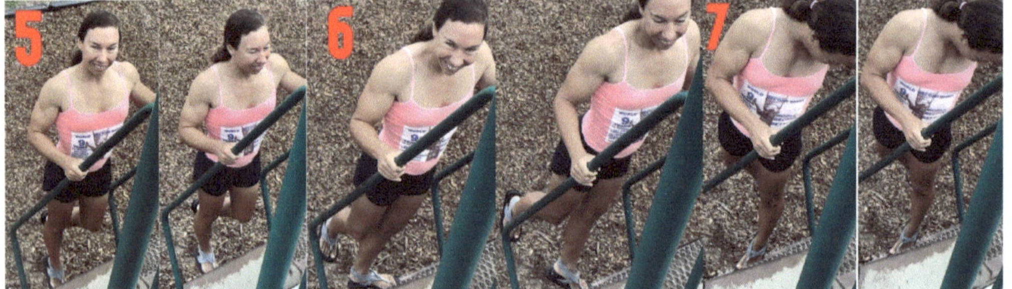

***This is an effective routine that can be part of your warn-up (before exercises or competition).**

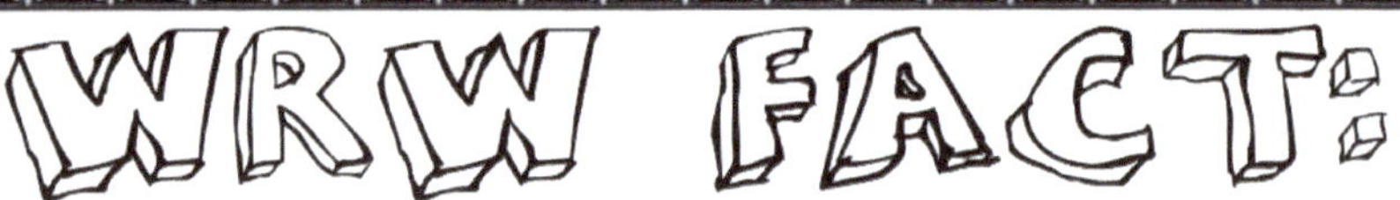

Alicia and her Team Awinningway hold Global Running Participation World Records. In 2016 Alicia and her team set the World Record for "Most Florida Runners Participating in a One Mile Cross Country Race for Global Running Day" with 6 participants. In 2017 Alicia and a group of runners throughout Clermont set the World Record for "Most Runners in Florida Completing Middle Distance Races for Global Running Day" with 29 runners.

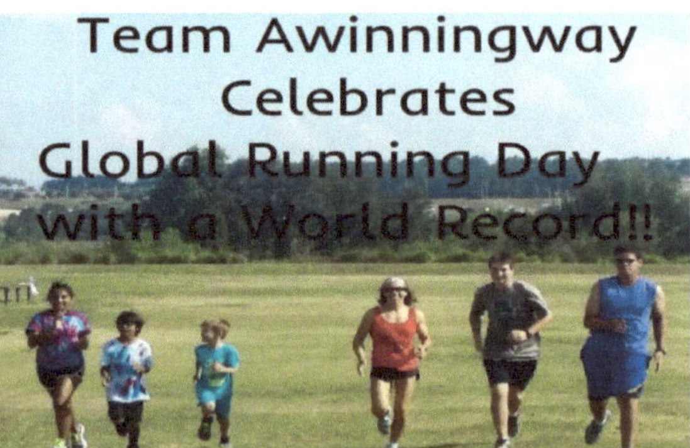

Top Times in Global Running Day Events:

2016 - Alicia Weber first set cross country course 1 mile record with 5:18.3. Also in 2016, Cody Warner (age 7) set youth mile record with 7:18.

2017 - Alicia was 11 seconds off her record on the one mile cross country course finishing in 5:29. She set the 800 meter cross country course record with 2:26. Also in 2017, Austin Englett (age 8) set the youth 800 meter cross country course record with his time of 3:10. The youngest participant to help set a Global Running Day World Record was age 2 completing one mile. Alicia trained the participants who set the course records.

2018 - Alicia lowered her 800 meter course record down to 2:20 on her favorite cross country course, which involves two small hills within a 0.25 mile grass circle.

3

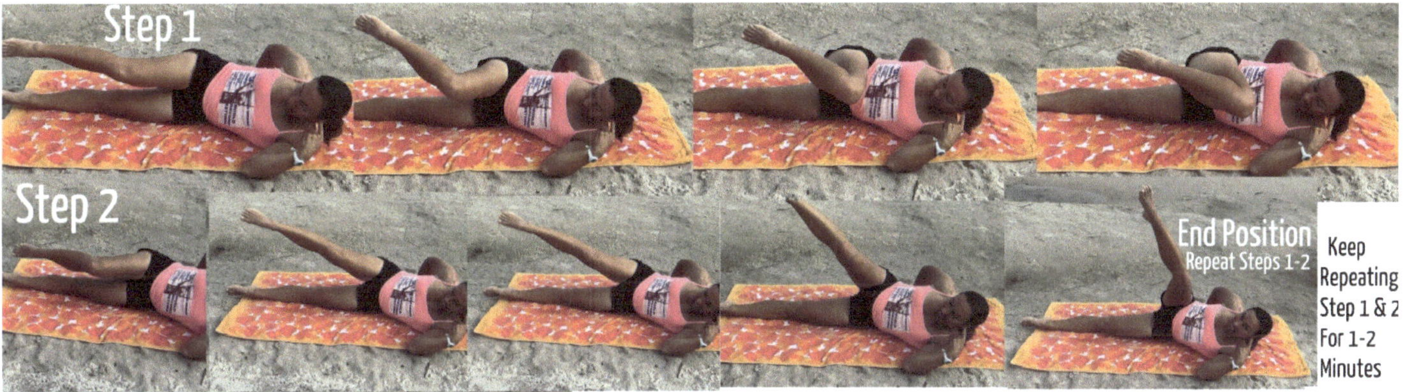

Alligator Lock Jaw (Keep moving at continuous Tempo Pace for 1-2 minutes following step 1 and 2).

Progression: Follow step 1 and 2 by beginning with a forward thrust till you get a firm end feel. Then, return leg straight down by other leg. Finally, drive leg straight up like making an alligator's mouth. If you do this at a good, steady pace, then you will begin to get a "burn" in 1-2 minutes (you want to feel the burn). After, 1-2 mins go into step 3. This final step known as the "alligator lock jaw" is when we will pulse the leg up slowly to try and open the alligator's mouth all the way. With the thighs burning, it can be hard to achieve. You end when mouth is almost open or all the way open. The burn achieved is what is building strength and tightening thigh.

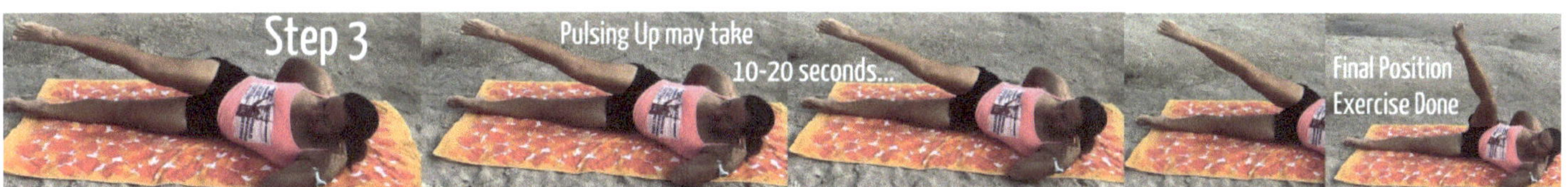

Goal: Feel the burn. Build stength in thighs, firm thighs, and stretch/strengthen low back.

Purpose: This is a great exercise for anyone looking to tighten and tone thighs quickly. This also builds ROM in hip joint.

WRW FACT:

RECORD SETTER℠

On December 1, 2013, Alicia set the world record for the "Fastest Consecutive 100 Meter Plyometric Alligator Pushups" for the second time with a time of 9:05 (completing 138 pushups). She first set the record on the same track in Las Vegas, NV, in 2012 where she considered the record the most intense record to set in the year 2012 in 12:10.75 (185 pushups) on 11/21/12.

THE RULES FOR THE 100 METER PLYOMETRIC ALLIGATOR PUSHUPS ARE AS FOLLOWS:

1. MUST MAINTAIN A PLANK AND KEEP LEGS STRAIGHT AND FEET TOETHER (EVEN IN HOP).
2. MUST HOP AFTER EACH PUSHUP.
3. MUST REACH ONE ARM OUT, WHILE OTHER ARM IS CLOSE TO BODY FOR PUSHUP.
4. ALTERNATE CLOSE ARM AND REACHING OUT ARM FOR PUSHUPS.

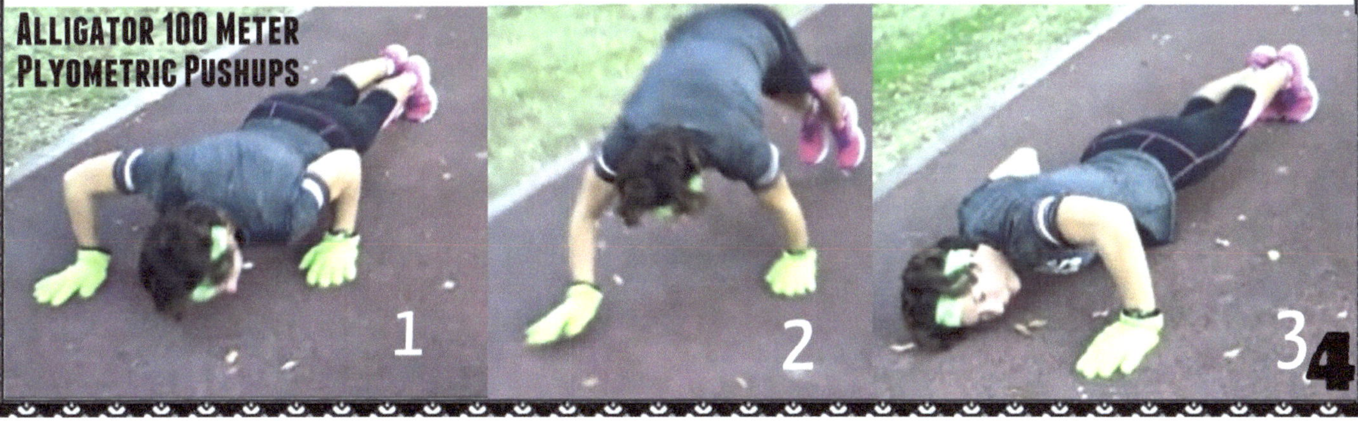

ALLIGATOR 100 METER PLYOMETRIC PUSHUPS

1   2   3   4

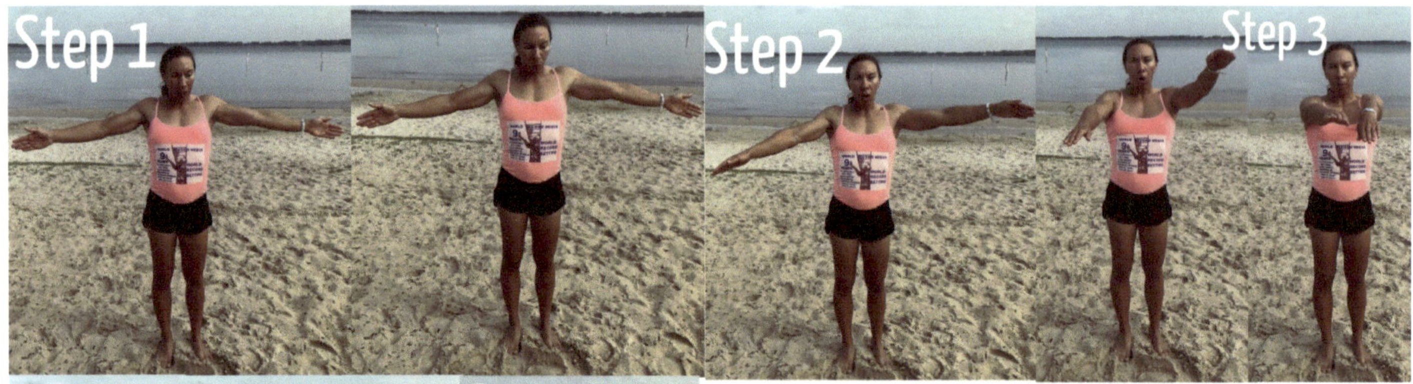

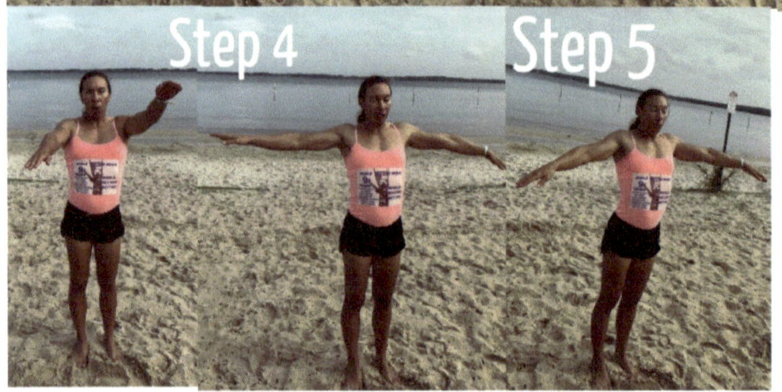

Around The World Arm Flaps (Move through 3 pulsing positions in 80 seconds.)

Purpose: This tightens and tones arms. Senior women have reported that they receive better "under arm" toning with arm flaps than they do with doing pushups. This is a winning routine to tighten and tone arms quickly.

Progressions: Pulse in 3 main positions by moving straight arms within 2 inches. Move at shoulder joint and not at the wrist. Do one set of 80 seconds. Rest and you can do 1-2 more sets.

Goal: Go through pulsing positions in following order:
Step 1 "airplane with wind on wings" pulse 20 seconds.
Step 2 pulse and move arms to center in 10 seconds.
Step 3 "arm bicycling" pulse 20 seconds.
Step 4 pulse and move arms back to sides in T in 10 seconds.
Step 5 "baby bird that can't fly out of nest" pulse 20 seconds.

WRW FACT:

Push-Up Hall of Fame
9 Push-Up World Champions

In January of 2012, Alicia became the first and only woman inducted into the Official Pushup Hall of Fame at www.facebook.com/TheOfficialPushUpHallOfFame

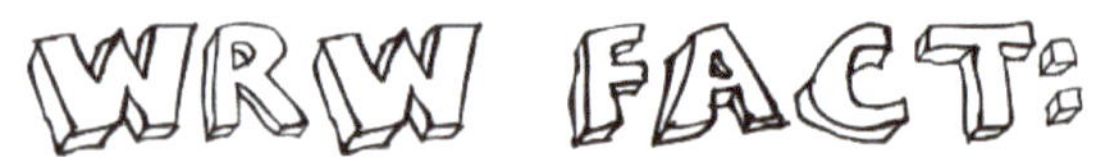

Here are some of Alicia's pushup world records:
1. Most consecutive shoulder-width grip pushups in 30 minutes (771) set on 3.22.17.
2. Most consecutive shoulder-width grip pushups in One hour (1,195) set on 2.10.18.
3. Most consecutive shoulder-width grip pushups in 15 minutes (484) set on 11.18.17.
4. Most consecutive shoulder-width grip pushups in 10 minutes (358) set on 11.18.17.
5. Most consecutive pushups in 3 minutes (167) set on 10.18.17.

*Must perform pushups on hard surface. Must keep legs no more than hip-width apart. Must bend arms to at least 90 degrees and return to extension.

RECORD SETTER

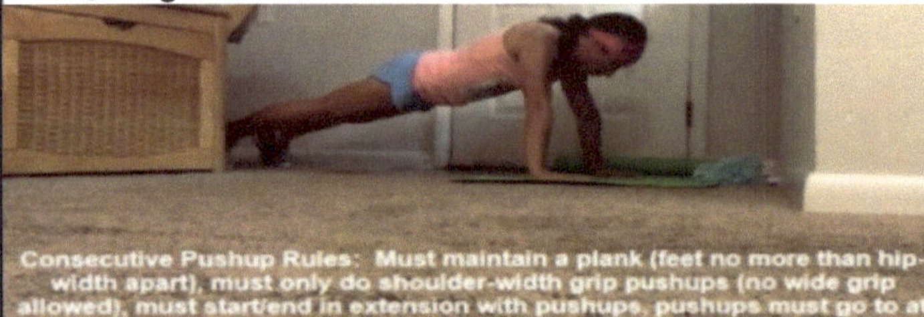

Consecutive Pushup Rules: Must maintain a plank (feet no more than hip-width apart), must only do shoulder-width grip pushups (no wide grip allowed), must start/end in extension with pushups, pushups must go to at least 90 degrees (parallel to ground).

On 11.18.17, Alicia competed in Florida's First SUP Drag Race. It was a very short all out sprint in Treasure Island. Alicia placed 3rd in prelims for the co-ed race and 4th in female only final. Later in the day, she broke the 10 and 15 minute consecutive pushup world records.

On 5.20.17, Alicia won her first Florida Cup Short Course Championship at St. Pete Beach, FL. She placed 1st woman overall in SUP surfboard class and 18th overall among all board classes and genders.

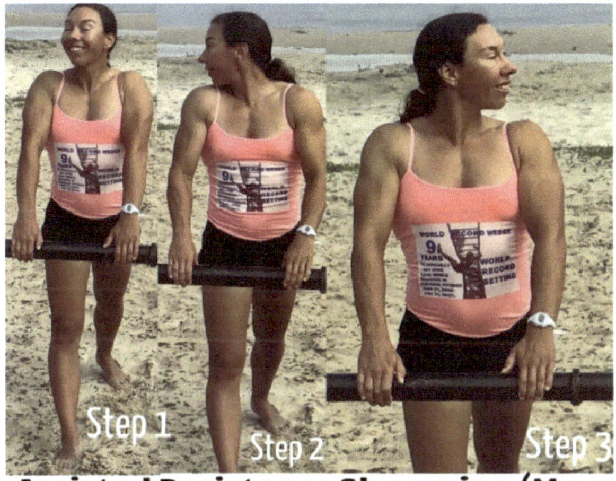

Roll Forward To Backward Shrugs.

Step 1 center position.

Step 2 shrugging and turning head slowly to right.

Step 3 shrugging and turning head slowly to left.

Purpose: Build ROM in shoulders and neck.
Break up tightness in neck and shoulders.
Loosen upper body to prepare for exercises
or reduce stiffness.

Assisted Resistance Shrugging (Move shoulders with head right to left s-l-o-w-l-y for 3 - 10 shrugs forward to back shrugs ABOVE and Backward to forward shrugs BELOW.)

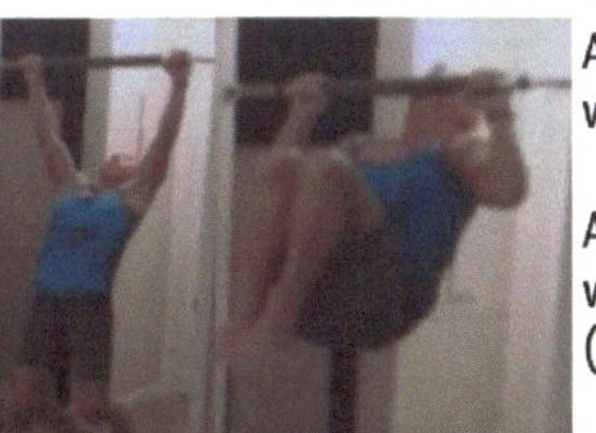

Roll Backward to Forward Shrugs.

Step 1 center position.

Step 2 shrugging and rolling shoulders forward, while turning head slowly to left.

Step 3 shrugging and rolling shoulders forward, while turning head slowly to right.

Purpose: Build ROM in shoulders and neck.
Stretch out back to prepare for upper body
exercises or to reduce stiffness.

Goal: Build ROM in neck and shoulders
and prevent upper body muscles
and neck from getting tight.

WRW FACT:

Alicia has set and re-set many world records for pull-ups, chin-ups, and rope climbing.

Highlighted below are Alicia's most challenging record categories to set and re-set based on length of preparation and level of difficulty to set and re-set.

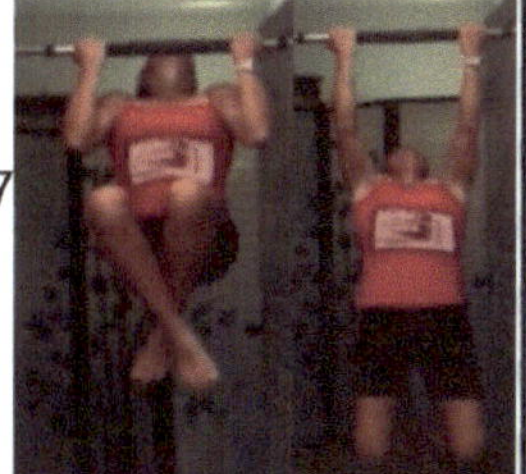

Alicia set world record for "Most Pull-ups in One Hour (palm-away grip)" on June 22, 2016 with 1,070 pull-ups. Must start in dead hang full-extension and take chin over bar = 1 rep.

Alicia set world record for "Most Shoulder-Width Grip Chin-Ups in 30 minutes" on Nov 7, 2017 with 502 reps all with only shoulder-width grip. Must start in dead hang full extension (palm toward you grip only) and take chin over bar=1 rep

*All records listed here are not allowed to use leg movements to help.

RECORD SETTER

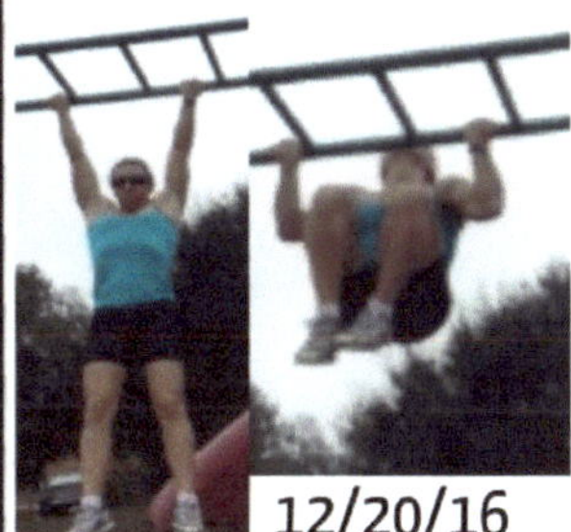

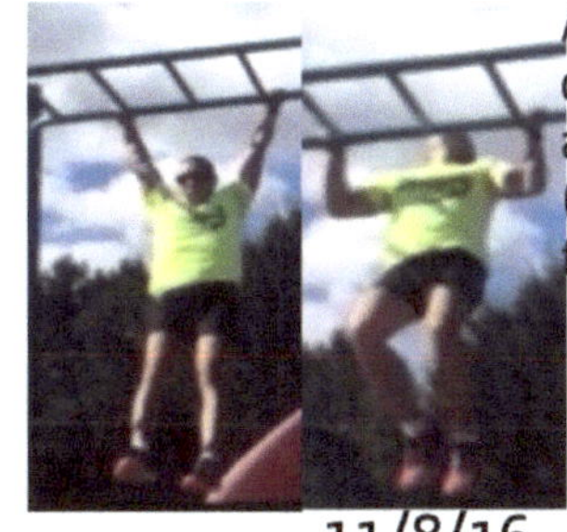

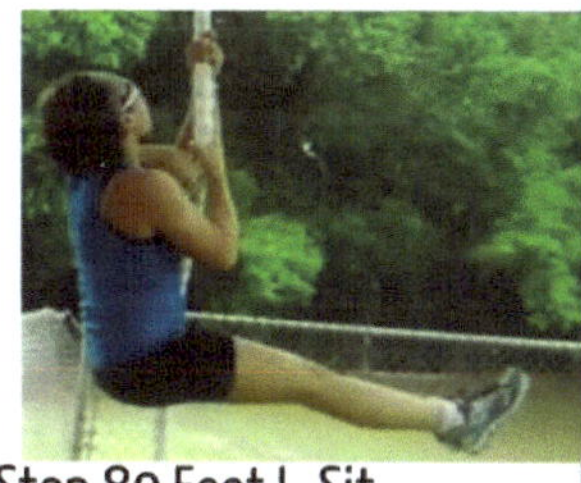

Alicia set both "Most Consecutive Strict Pull-Ups on a Thick Bar (measuring at least 6 inches around)" and "Most Consecutive Strict Chin-Ups on a thick bar (measuring 6 inches around)" with 59 reps for both records in fall 2016.

*Each rep must be completed in max 6 seconds for reps to be consecutive.

Alicia set world record for "Fastest Non-Stop 80 Feet L-Sit Rope Climb" in 48.91 seconds on June 13, 2015. She must start in sitting position and never touch ground during L-sit climb.

12/20/16
Thick Grip Chin-Ups

11/8/16
Thick Grip Pull-Ups

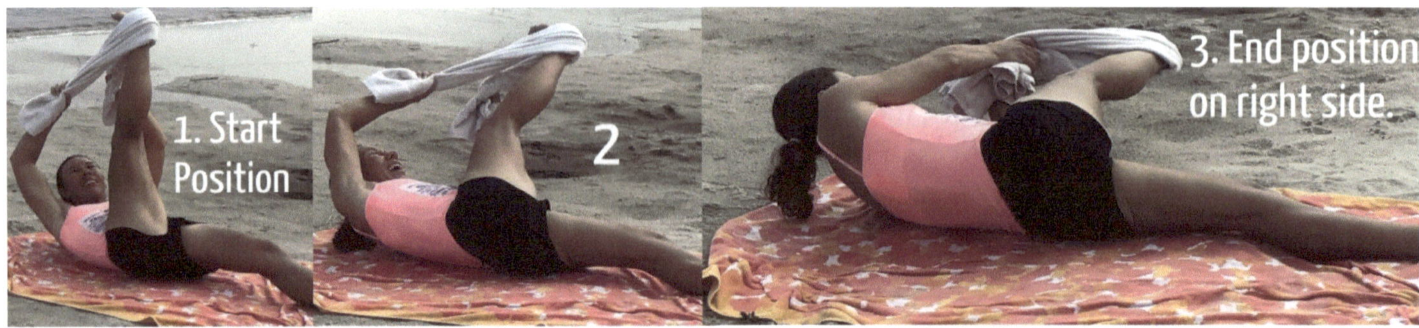

Resistance Towel Leg Stretch

Purpose: This stretch has been known to get rid of leg pains and also get rid of various leg problems that doctors were unable to diagnose.

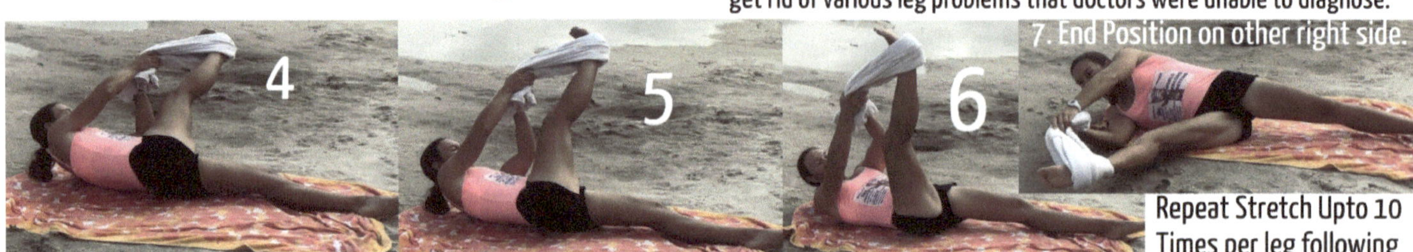

Goal: Keep both legs straight (non-moving leg held vertical), while moving leg will rotate and goal is to make a 90 degree angle in both end positions (3 and 7). Do equal reps on both legs with the towel resistance.

Repeat Stretch Upto 10 Times per leg following pictures 1-7. Rotate moving leg slowly and hold end positions 3 and 7 for at least 3 seconds. Keep non-moving leg straight and vertical.

WORKING TOWARD WORLD RECORDS...

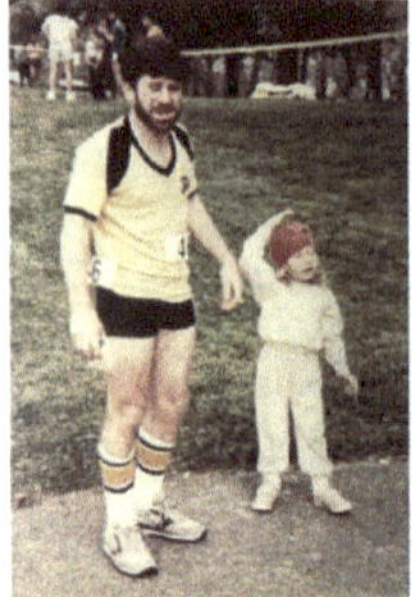

Alicia (age 4) inspired to become a determined athlete after watching her dad compete in the 1984 North Park .PA Triathlon.

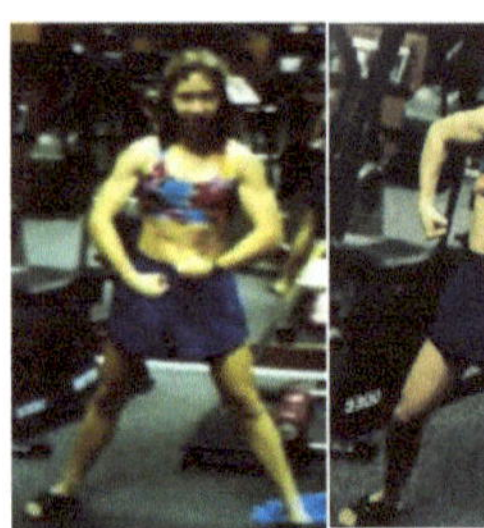

Alicia at age 13 in training (just before setting a bunch of all time physical fitness test records at South Park Middle School).

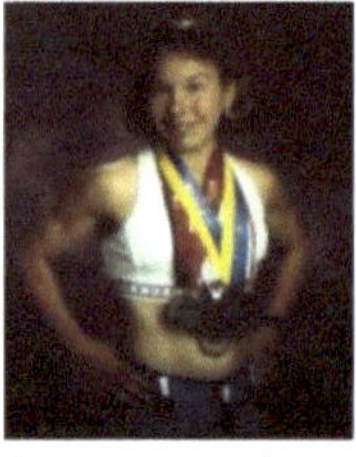

Alicia age 17 with 7 medals from National Championships.

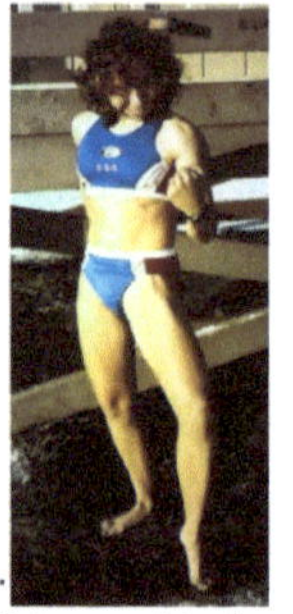

Alicia age 24 after winning North American Nova Fitness Championship and setting 5 North American Records (1st out of men and women).

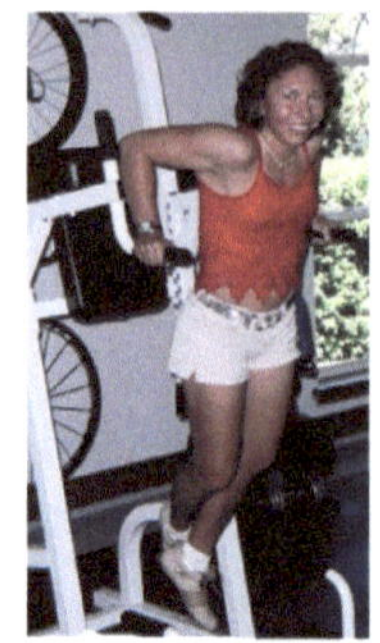

Alicia age 27 after setting her first official world record with 75 consecutive bar dips in 5 Minutes in 2008. She now holds the world record with 133 set in 2015.

RECORD SETTER™

World Record Weber Progressions

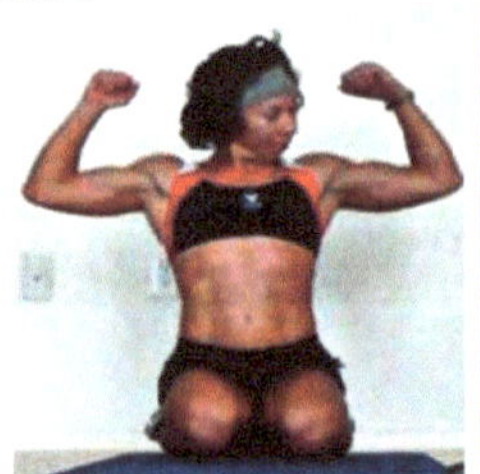

2009
After Setting 20 World Records

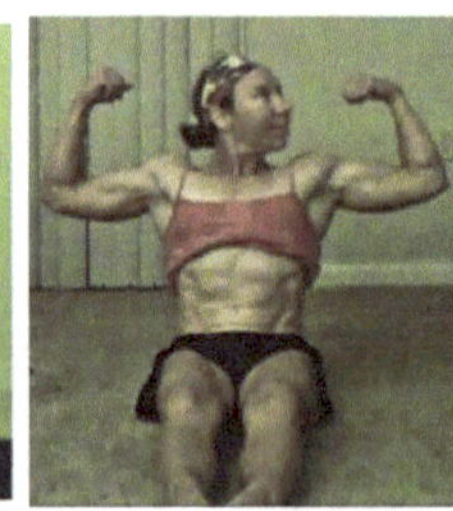

2011
After Setting Over 40 World Records

2016
Setting over 800 World Records.

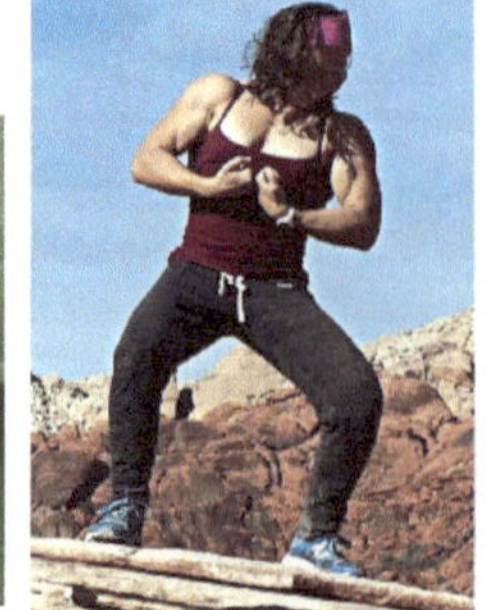

2018 Setting Over 1,000 World Records.

7

Leg Balance and Stability Strengtheners

(TOP) Eyes Shut Thrust Lunges

Purpose: Build feet and leg strength, balance, and stabilty. Helps prevent ankle sprains/strains.

Goal: Keep eyes shut. Begin with one leg held straight back. Thrust front leg to a firm end feel to work hip flexors and build ROM. Set thrusting leg down with 70-90 degree bend (keeping knee over the heel). This is a slow moving exercise and go for at least 10 reps alternating lunge legs.

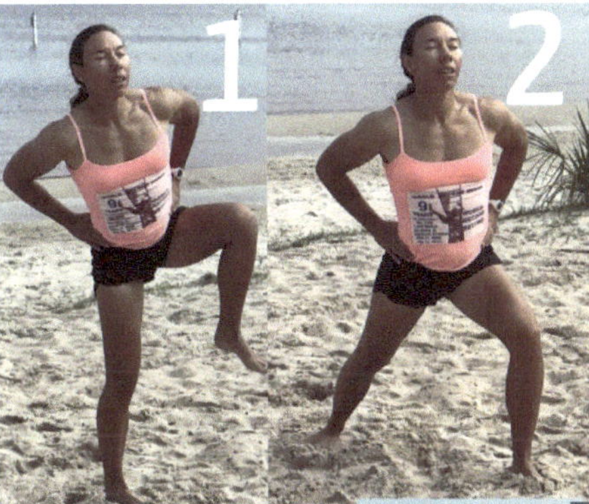

(Center) Thrust Lunge with Arms Swinging (follow description for TOP exercise with eyes open).

Goal: Go into a lunge and swing arms back and forth at 90 dgrees 2-4 times per lunge.
Do at least 10 lunges. The arm swinging is aggressive with a straight back and this builds core strength.

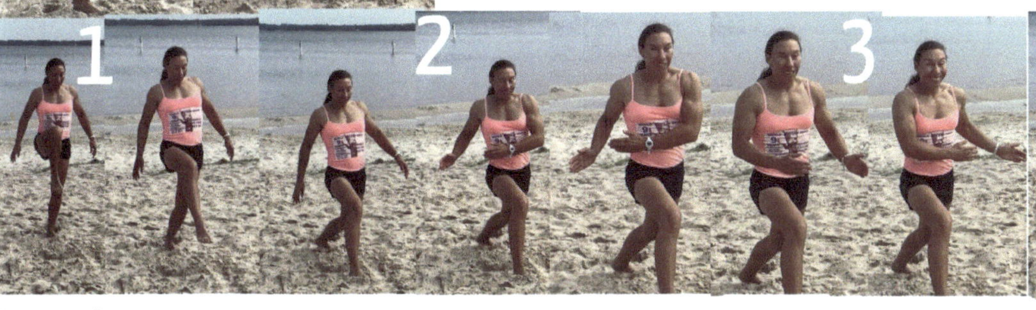
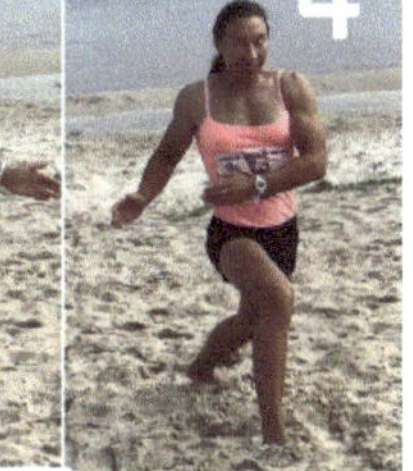

(Bottom) Windshield Wipers for Knee Strengthening

Purpose: Builds knee strength and stability. It works muscles, ligaments, and tendons around knee to help stabiliize it

Goal: Balance and keep front leg bent with knee held over heel. Keep back leg (moving leg) straight. Invert back straight leg then move it out to wide stance. Objective is to keep (non-moving) leg around knee stabile. Do 5-10 windshield wiper reps per leg. One windshield wiper is out and back.

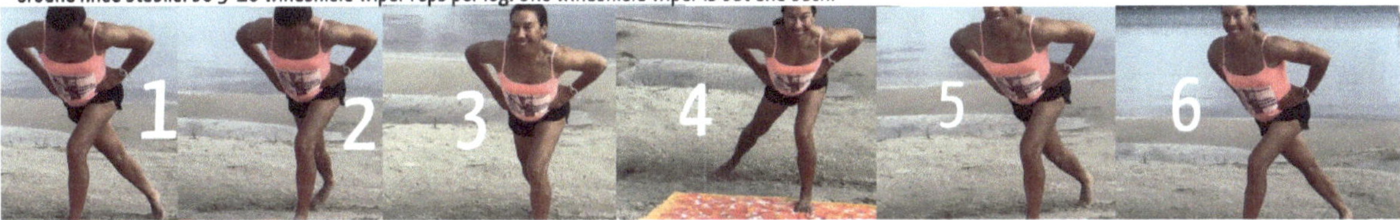

Picture Shows
1 rep of a
Windshield Wiper.

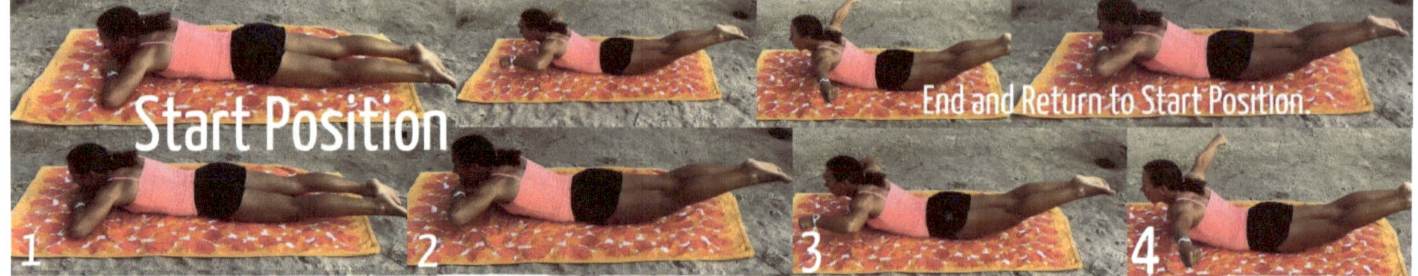

Core Strengtheners and Stretchers

Above Exercise is Known as the "Backup" and the best exercise to strengthen back and stop back pain.

Goal: Do one set of upto 10 slow reps in 2 minutes.

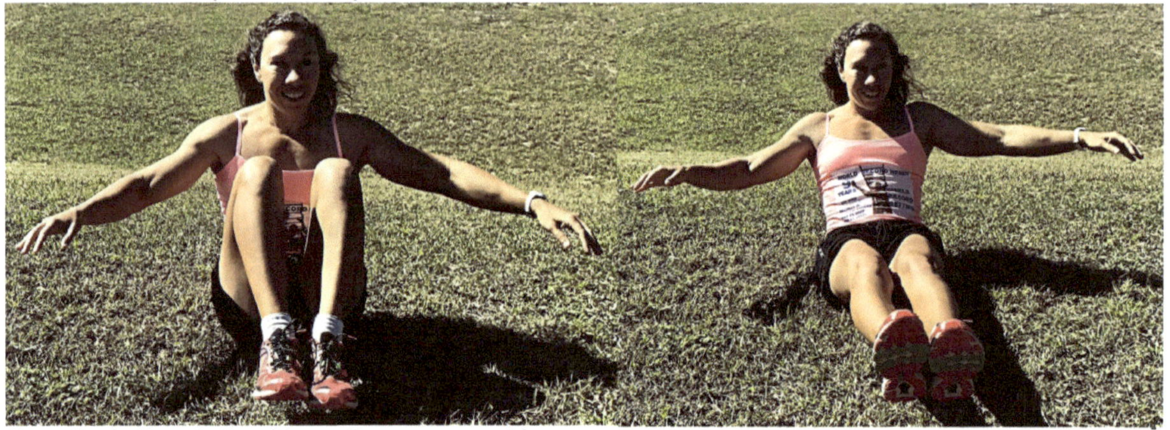

Knee Tuck Step 1: Bend Legs, Keep arms at sides, and Keep back upright.

Knee Tuck Step 2: Balance the body upright. Stretch legs out and keep feet from touching the ground.

The "Knee Tuck" shown here is the best all around core exercise and it works balance too.

Goal: Try to do one rep of a knee tuck in max 3 seconds. Stay balanced and see how many you can do in two minutes or until failure.

WRW FACT:

Alicia enjoys challenging herself and clients in core challengings. Below are some of her records and client records.

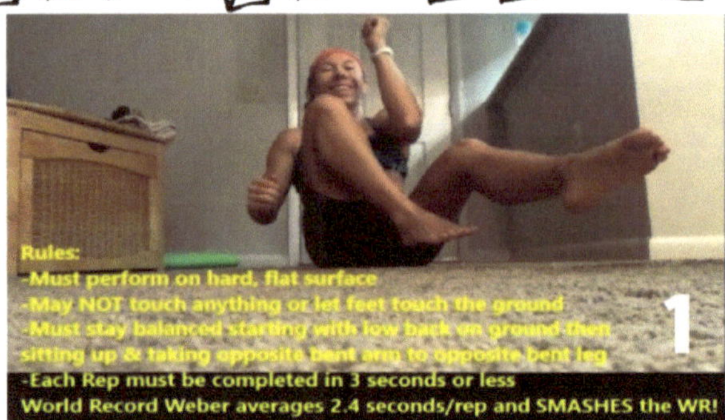

1. Alicia set world record for "Most Consecutive Sprinter Situps" with 410 reps on August 12, 2017.

2. On September 6, 2017 Alicia re-set the "Consecutive Knee Tuck" world record for the 13th time when she did 1,157 reps.

3. Alicia's client, Bonnie Jean, holds the world record for "Most Consecutive Knee Tucks by a Female over 60 Years Old" with 96 reps set on December 17, 2012.

4. Alicia set world record for "Longest Cadence Back-Up Exercise" where she had to do 30 back-ups every minute till failure. The record is 21 minutes set on June 24, 2012.

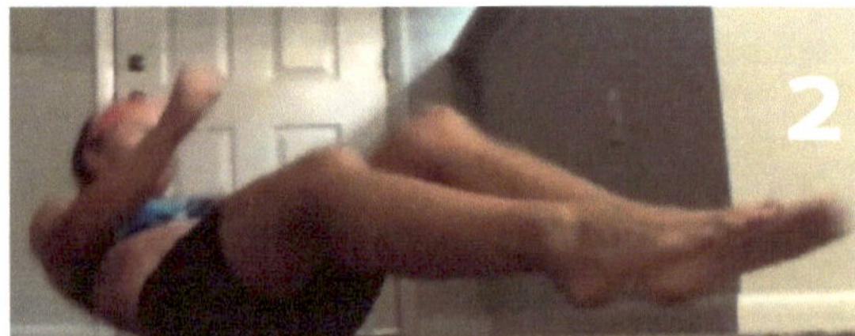

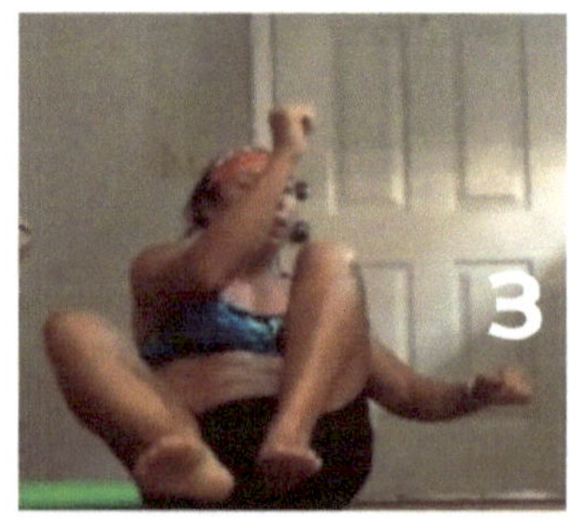

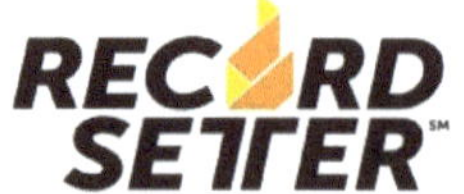

Pictures demonstrate the steps in doing the Sprinter Situp. In Step 2, keep feet and upper back off the ground.

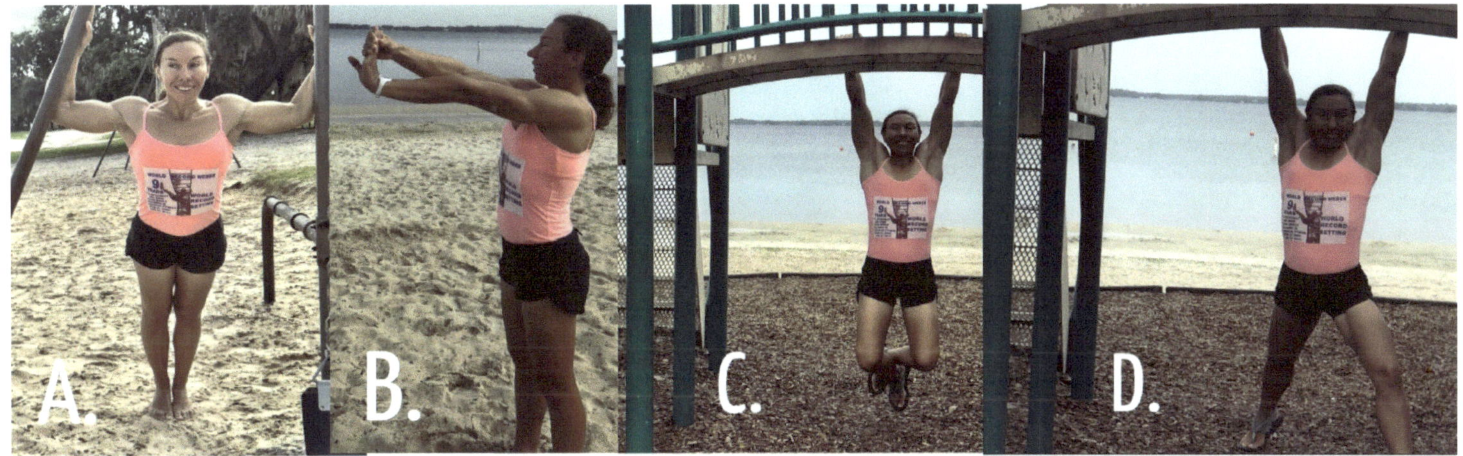

Well-Rounded Stretch n' Strengthen kit for Small Muscles (Do one rep of each move. Hangs/Holds are a minimum of 10-20 seconds or until failure.)

A. Doorway Stretch for shoulders, chest, and upper back   E. Finger Pilates to loosen fingers
B. Wrist Stretch to loosen wrist and forearm
C. Hanging Stretch to stretch entire upper-body
D. Hanging Lunge Stretch to open up hips and upper and lower body

Purpose: Each move is held in static position except E. Finger Pilates (where you take 2 fingers and take turns pulling and stretchin each finger top to bottom). These moves are known to heal strains and tendonitis and prevent injuries by strengthening small muscles.

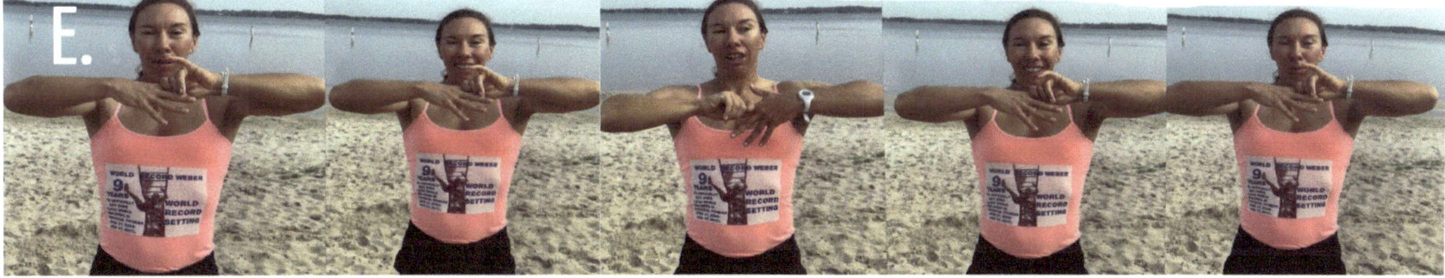

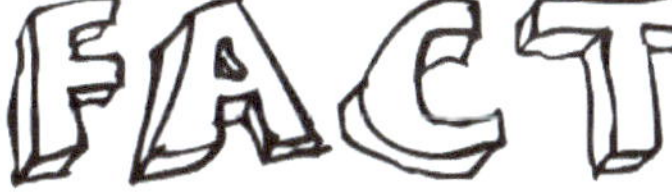

Alicia developed a new record category and sport known as "Archery Fitness" events back in 2013. She has an archery fitness league, which trains and competes in 2 championships a year. Below is her winningest team in Archery Fitness Sport History!

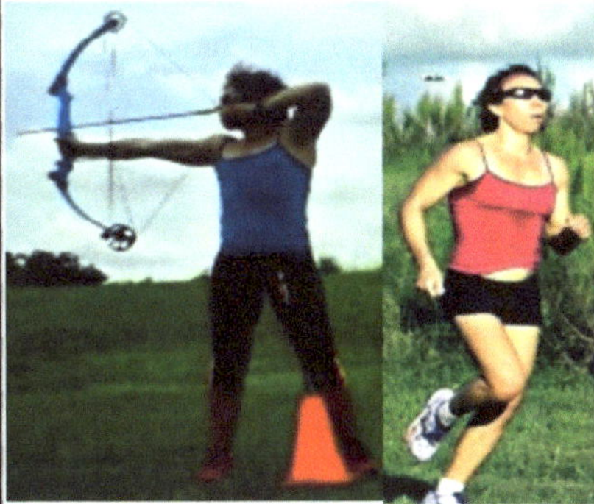

Alicia created a variety of exercise and archery record categories, but one of her favorite categories is combining speed cross country running with short distance speed shooting for fastest bullseye at 10 yards. The following are some of her records:

1. Fastest Time to perform a cross country 400 meter dash with a 10 yard Archery Bullseye (1:20.31) set on October 26, 2015.

2. Fastest Time to perform a 1500 meter cross country run with a 10 yard Archery Bullseye (5:26.35) on May 6, 2014.

3. Fastest time to perform a cross country half mile run with a 10 yard archery bullseye (2:52.30) on June 24, 2015.

Alicia only competes and sets records in the toughest type of archery without use of sighting devices (Barebow Category Archery).

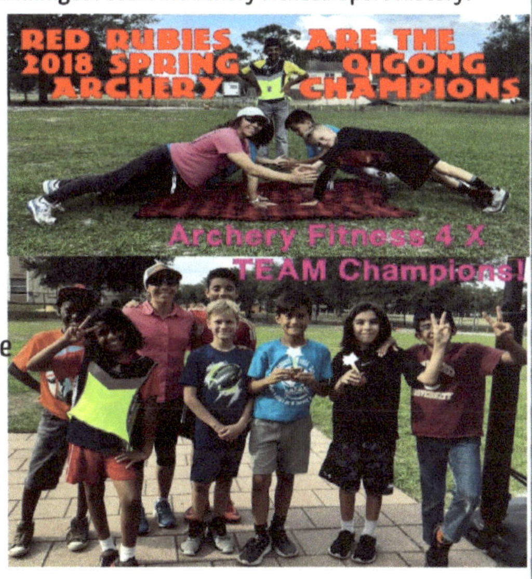

Alicia Weber's Archery Fitness League only competes in Barebow Category Archery.
AliciaWeber.com/archery

RECORD SETTER™

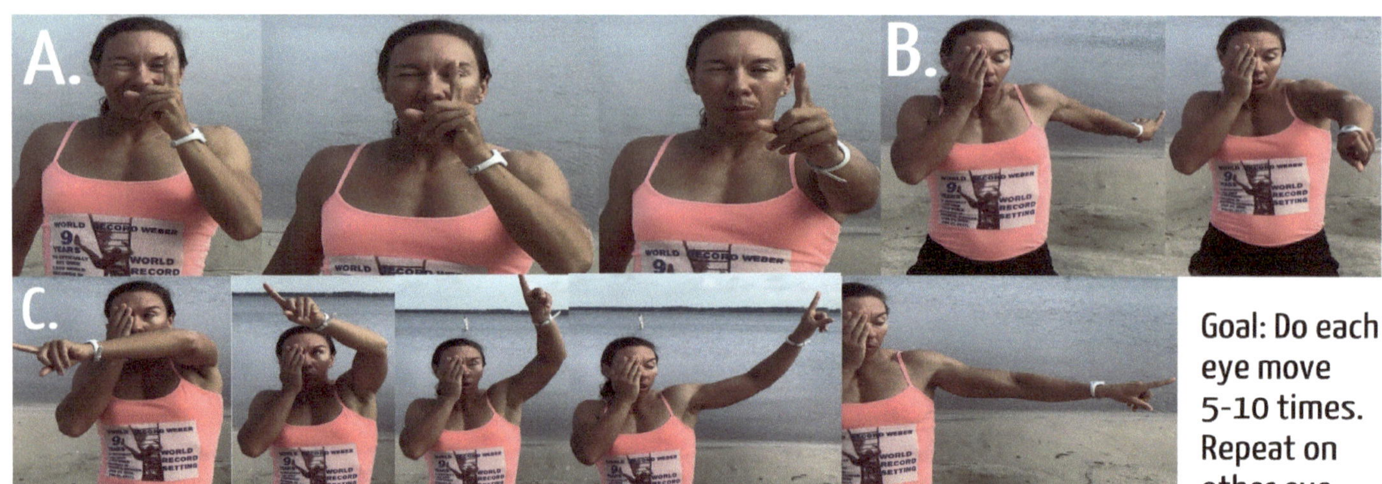

Eye Strengthening Exercises (Do each exercise as often as needed during week. One set of 5-10 reps is very effective.)

A. One Eye open stretch with finger moving toward eye and away
B. Head Straight Eye look back to see finger to build peripheral vision
C. Eye Follow Finger Circles

Purpose: Each eye exercise works to keep eyes sharp.

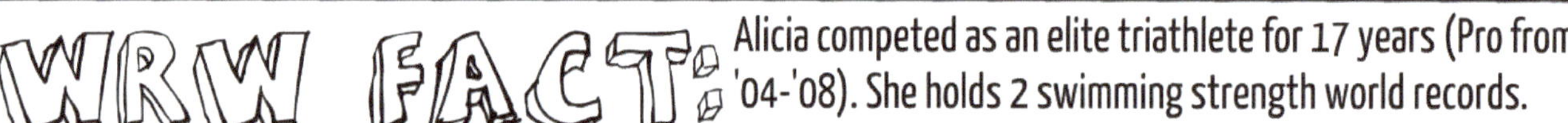

Alicia competed as an elite triathlete for 17 years (Pro from '04-'08). She holds 2 swimming strength world records.

Alicia became CPR/Lifeguard Certified back in high school. Her first job at age 17 was lifeguarding in PA.

Below demo for tricep "Triangle" Pushups.

Alicia set the world record in 50 meter pool for the "Fastest time to perform 100 consecutive Tricep "Triangle" Pushups with a 100 meter freestyle swim" with 5:41.35 on June 18, 2012.

*She had to start swim from wall start in both records(no diving or jumping start). Pushups always completed before swim.

Alicia set world record for "Fastest time to perform 200 consecutive pushups and a 200 meter freestyle swim" with 7:45.45 on September 6, 2015. This record can be set in short sized pool.

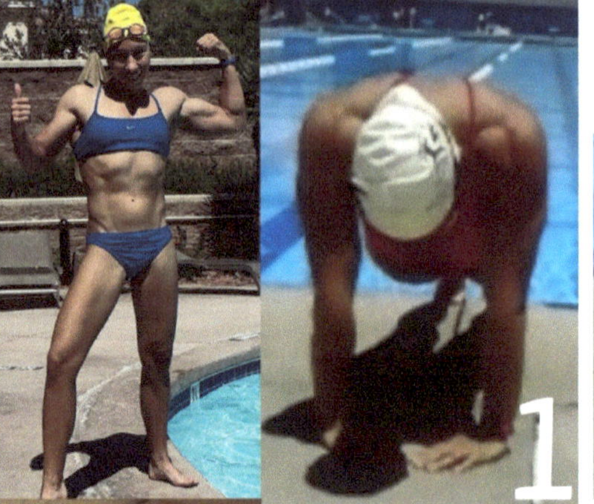

Alicia has been teaching swimming and aquatic training for over 20 years. She can teach someone how to swim in 3 lessons.

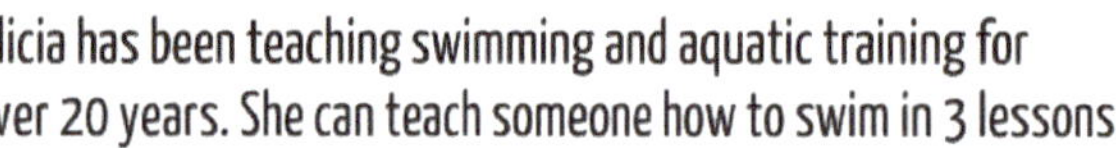

Alicia was undefeated Junior (U20) Sprint Triathlete and placed in Top 10 in sprints with open women. She made her first world team in Junior ITU Olympic Distance Triathlon at age 19. She represented US in Perth, Australia, for the 2000 ITU Olympic Distance Triathlon. As a pro, her best place was 9th in Nation at 2008 ITU Sprint National Championship for U30 triathletes. In 2009, she placed 14th in nation among men and women in Open Water Swimming 1 Mile National Championship. Her best time for the ocean 1 mile swim is 20:27.

11

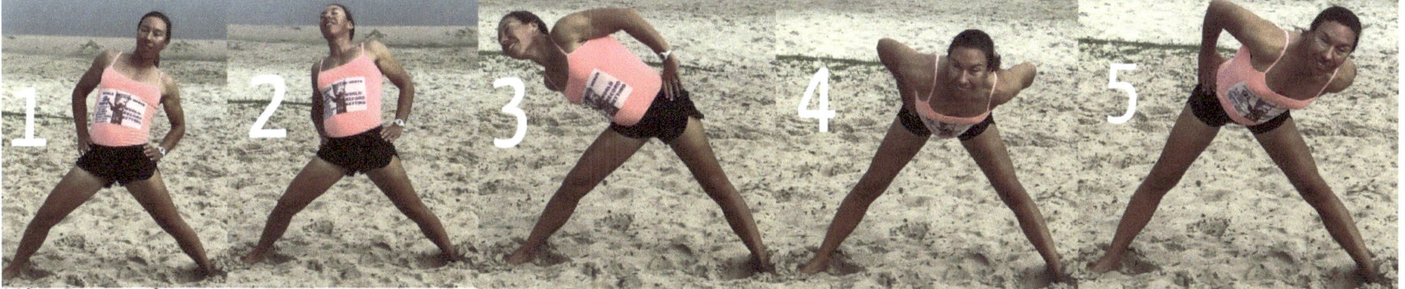

Hip Rotations
Goal: 5-10 slow circles in one direction. Repeat in other direction. Start forward, roll back, and roll center = 1 circle

Hip Swings

Goal: 5-10 slow hip swings. Keep back straight. Start with inverting moving leg. Then, swing leg out and pause at a firm end feel. Move leg back to start position =1 rep

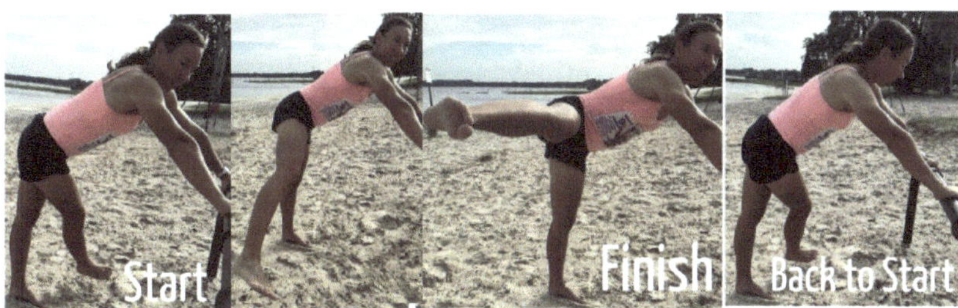

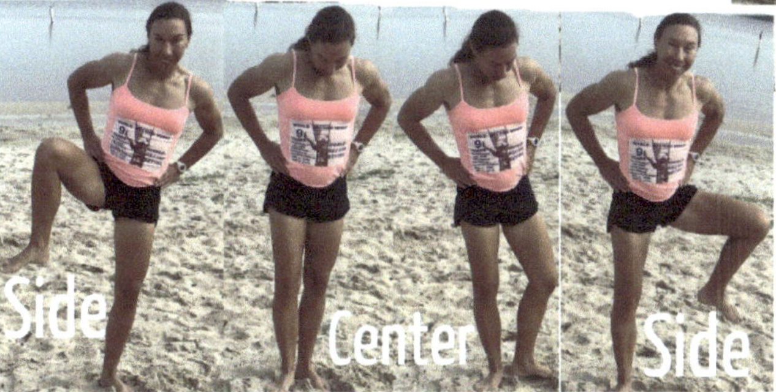

Standing Spiderman
Goal: Form a 90 degree angle with feet.
Lift one leg to side till a firm end feel, then repeat other leg for 5-10 reps.

Purpose: The following 3 stretches open up the hips to prevent injury and increase flexibility. They target the 3 angles of the hip joint.

Hip Stretches

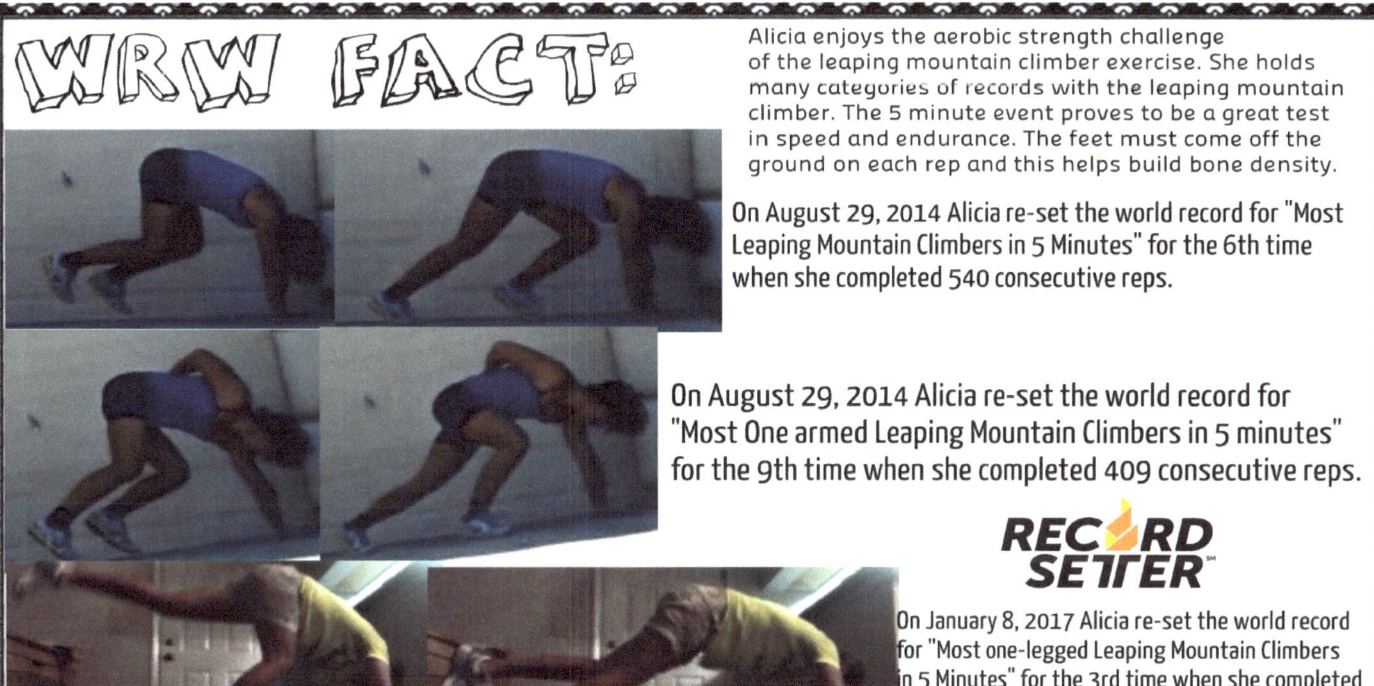

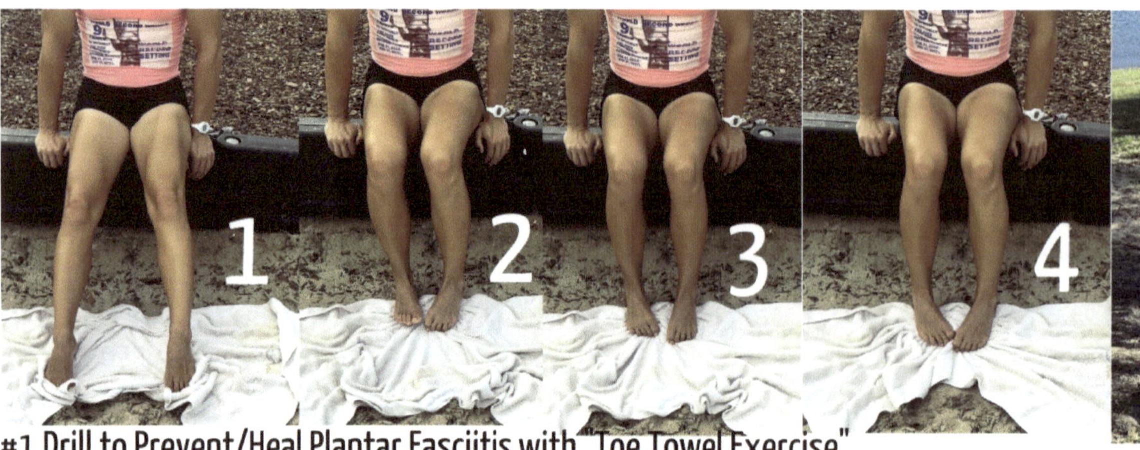

#1 Drill to Prevent/Heal Plantar Fasciitis with "Toe Towel Exercise"

Goal: Keep heel on ground and use toes to spread out towel (step 1), then grab/squeeze towel together (step 4). Do upto 10 reps of Step 1-4 once to 3 times a day to heal plantar fasciitis.

(ABOVE) Achilles Tendon and Plantar Fascia 30 second stretch (each foot hold these positions).

Lower Body Injury Prevention Drills

#1 Drill to Strengthen Deep Hip Muscles to maintain good posture and a straight waistline when walking/running (no hip drop).

Forward Walking Hip Swing Drill - do 10 Steps.

Backward Walking Hip Swing Drill - do 10 steps.

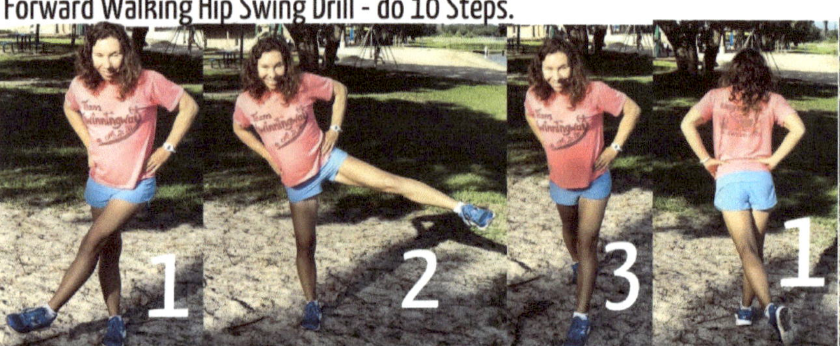

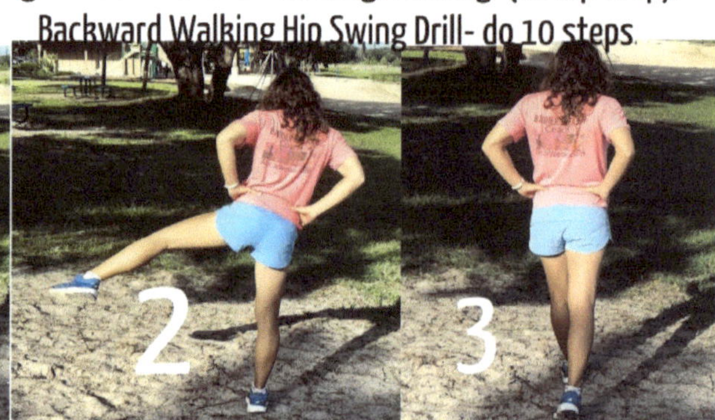

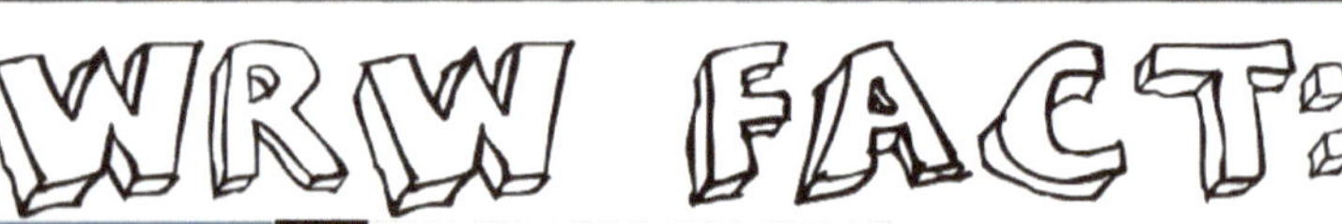

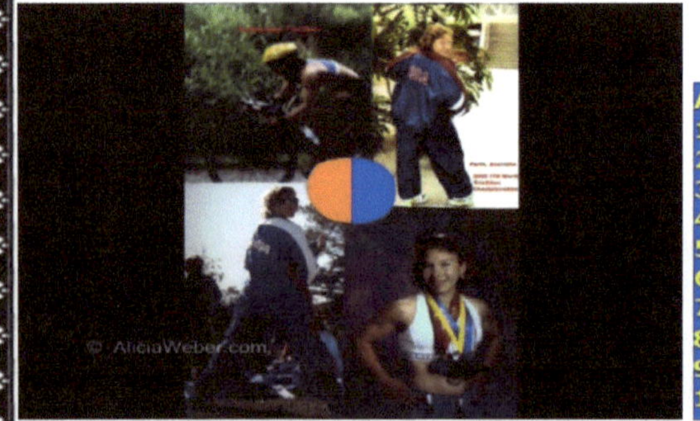

WRW FACT:

Striving for "wellness" means striving to be well-rounded. With over 650 muscles in the body, you need to try a lot of moves and new moves to keep everything strong + healthy! Alicia strives to set new records, re-set records, and work on many sports to challenge the mind and body.

On June 13-14, 2009, Alicia competed in a rare championship double. She first competed in State Championship for Sprint Kayak taking a gold (500m) and silver (200m) in Lakeland. Then, she went to Ft. Myers to compete in one mile Open Water Swimming Nationals where she placed 14th overall out of men and women.

In December of 2009, Alicia completed a year-long challenge of competing on the Elite level in the most individual sports. She had to compete in at least one National Championship or World Championship. An elite athlete is a competitor who competes for overall titles in their gender.

Alicia exceeded the record requirements as she competed in a National Championship for Open Water Swimming AND a World Championship for XTERRA Half-Marathon Running.

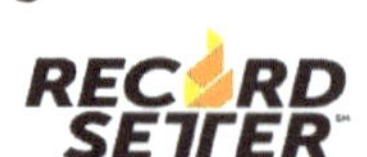

Alicia holds world record for "Most Sports Competed in at Elite Level in One Year" with 10 sports.

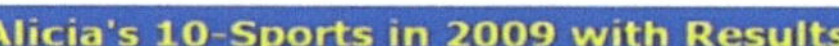

Alicia's 10-Sports in 2009 with Results
1. Mountain Running 40th in World
2. Trail Running 3rd in Southeast
3. Cross Country Running Runner-Up
4. Road Running 1 win
5. Triathlon 11th Elite in Southeast
6. Sprint Kayaking State Champ
7. Open Water Swimming 14th in Nation
8. Stand Up Paddle Boarding Runner-Up
9. Indoor Rowing 1 win
10. Exercise Challenges 8 World Records set

Alicia inducted 4 individuals (2 kids and 2 adults) and one class into her first year of her Hall of Fame in 2017. The inductees were chosen based on demonstrating a well-rounded wellness-mindset, striving for excellence, and contributing top performances for Team Awinningway. The inductees also show greatness by having longevity in sports, versatility, and consistency in performances.

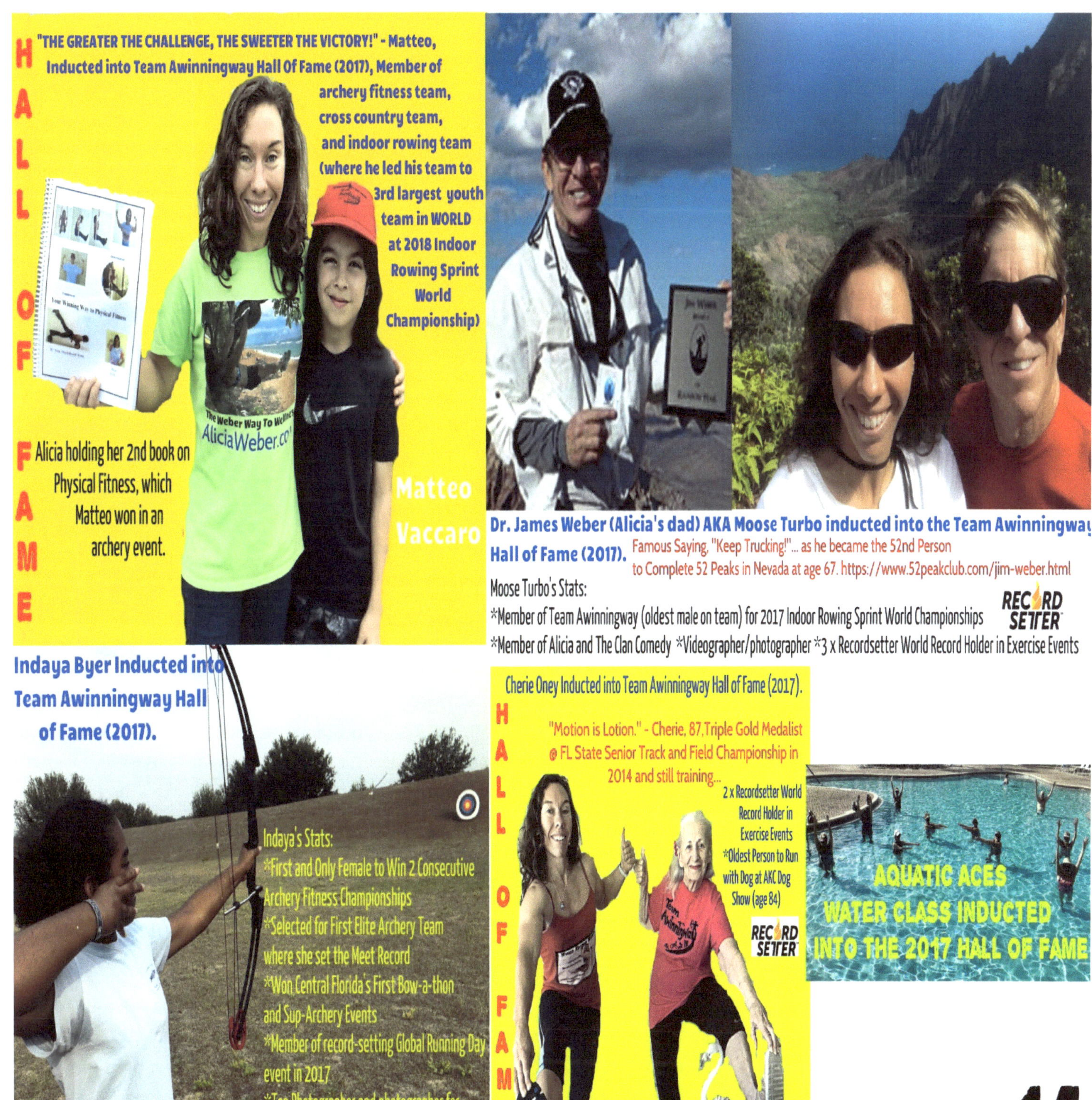

<u>**Alicia Weber's Aquatic Study on Building Bone Density (January 1, 2017-May 31, 2018)**</u>

Intro: Alicia Weber conducted a 1+ year study on her Hall of Fame Aquatic Aces to see if they could improve their bone density and reverse osteopenia through a new exercise routine Alicia developed known as "Aerobic Strength Planks" AKA "WRW Bone Density Builders" applied in their aquatic exercise class.

Background: It's a fact based on study results that *lack* of exercise leads to cognitive decline, dementia, and Alzheimer's disease. Studies show that the hippocampal volume decreases by 1-2% annually in adulthood. The only known way to reverse cognitive decline and increase hippocampal volume is through moderate exercise with resistance training as discovered in the following studies: 1. Exercise Increases Size of Hippocampus and Improves Memory (http://www.pnas.org/content/108/7/3017) 2. A Review of the Effects of Physical Activity and Exercise on Cognitive and Brain Functions in Older Adults (https://www.ncbi.nlm.nih.gov/pmc/articles/PMC3786463/). The studies found that the greater improvements in aerobic fitness (V02max) are associated with greater increase in hippocampal volume. Studies involving aquatic training show greater improvements in multi-tasking abilities and attentional control functions when compared to other forms of aerobic exercise. *Side Note: The Aquatic Aces do undergo a Total Mind + Body Workout where they have brain challenges regularly. Some of the Aquatic Aces were tested by their doctor in a mind test (testing cognitive function) and they passed with flying colors.*

Alicia's Study on Aquatic Aces: The Aquatic Aces consisted of a core group of 20 individuals ages 70-85 in Clermont, Florida (one male and the rest were female). They all have been doing water exercise for years and call aquatic exercise their main source of exercise. In this time frame, the individuals focused on mastering the new aquatic exercise routine and no changes were made to their nutrition and diet. Alicia only recommended that the Aquatic Aces take 200-500 milligrams of magnesium a day or eat a handful of walnuts (for magnesium) several times a week. Additionally, Alicia recommended eating bananas and/or taking Dr. Sinatra's Electrolyte PLUS for proper electrolytes, especially during hottest months.

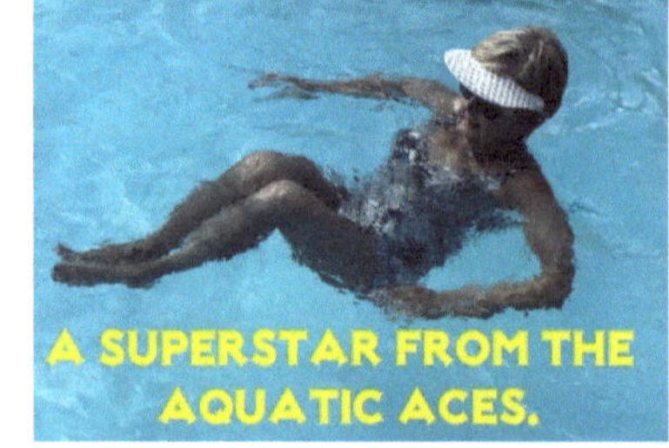

Alicia's Study Stats: Of the 20 individuals, 7-14 participants came on average to each class held three times a week for one hour. Classes were held on non-consecutive days to have rest days in between them. The classes averaged low-medium intensity with occasional high intensity bouts. However, starting from Feb-May 2018 two classes were low-medium intensity for one hour and the last class each week became a 45 minute high-intensity aquatic training class. All three weekly classes involved Alicia's new "Aerobic Strength Plank" exercises. In January 2017, participants began doing only 3-5 minutes of "Aerobic Strength Plank" exercises per class and they built up to a maximum of 20 minutes doing consecutive "Aerobic Strength Plank" exercises. The average class does 30-40 minutes of continuous cardio with 8 minutes of "Aerobic Strength Plank" exercises.

Alicia's Study Results: After the first month, the Aquatic Aces felt a significant increase in leg strength and flexibility i.e. improved walking (especially walking upstairs) and improved hip height to step up into a big van or truck. As time went on, other results were reported including but not limited to increased energy, reduced edema and inflammation in feet and legs, greater ability to walk longer distances, increased overall strength, improved balance and gait, better posture, and improved endurance. Finally, it was time to get the real results as the one year marked arrived---The Aquatic Aces got checked by their doctor and took a bone density test. All of the Aquatic Aces that received their checkups got a clean bill of health and they all improved bone density even by a small fraction. Some improved bone density more than others and some reversed osteopenia. At the conclusion of the study, the Aquatic Aces stated in agreement, "We can't imagine how we would be, if we were not doing this regular aquatic program."

Conclusion: The "Aerobic Strength Planks" AKA "WRW Bone Density Builder" exercises work to improve bone density, reverse osteopenia, and prevent osteoporosis.

15

WRW Bone Density Builders AKA Aerobic Strength Planks (Plank Jack Series)

Goal: Stimulate fast twitch muscle fibers, quick reaction time, strength, and flexibility.

Progressions: Complete in any order...modified or advanced depending on fitness level. Remember, Aquatic Aces only did Plank Jacks in shallow pool using wall (head out of water). You may do on land by kitchen counter. Alicia only does the advanced moves in training. Advanced start with just a few reps. Proper form is key. Modified go by time...

Aquatic Aces would do ony 1 set for 30 seconds to 2 minutes per exercise. NOTE: Arms are Straight in ALL exercises.

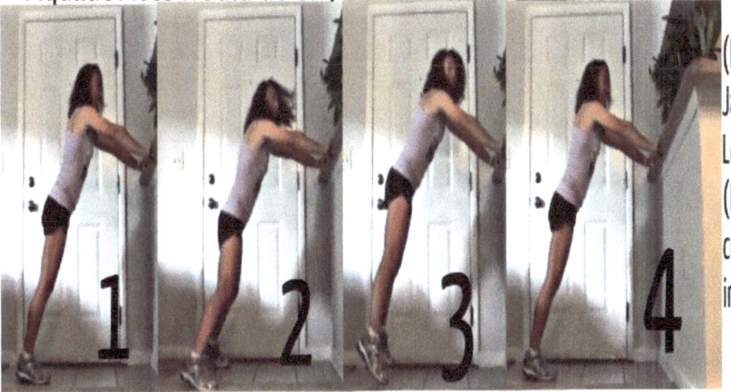

(L) 1-4 Standard Plank Jack at wall Diagonal Legs out hip-width jump in.
(R) Continue 5-8 Jump center legs move out and in at least once for a rep.

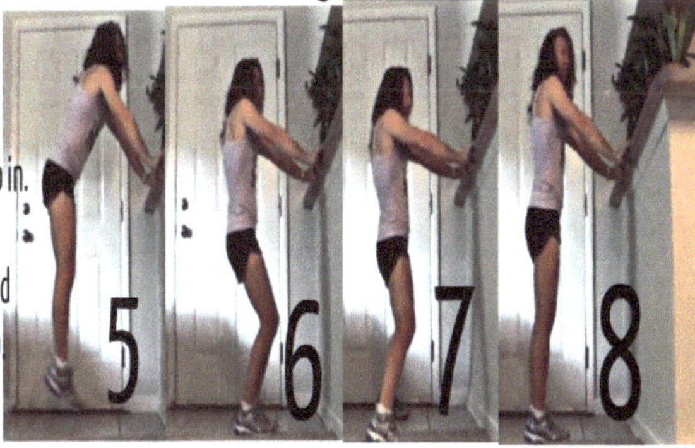

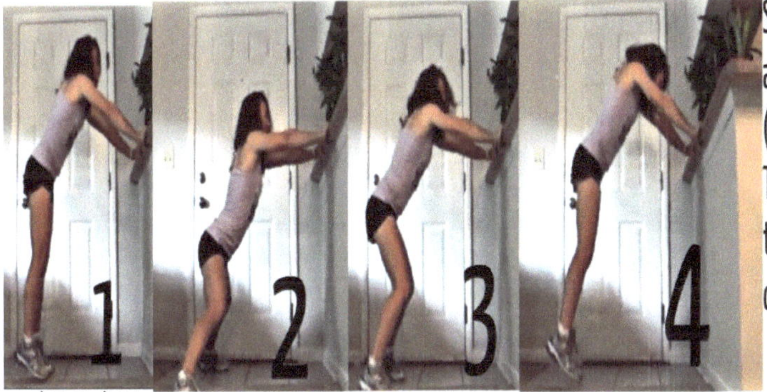

(L) Flexibility Plank Jack

Stay diagonal and jump wide out (more than 3 feet). Take 3 Small jumps to return feet center =1 rep

(BELOW) Advanced Plank Jacks

1-3 Stay in plank and jump feet apart 2-3 feet. Then, return center =1 rep
4-8 Jump Center and jump feet apart 2-3 feet. Then, return center =1 rep
End back in plank (8).

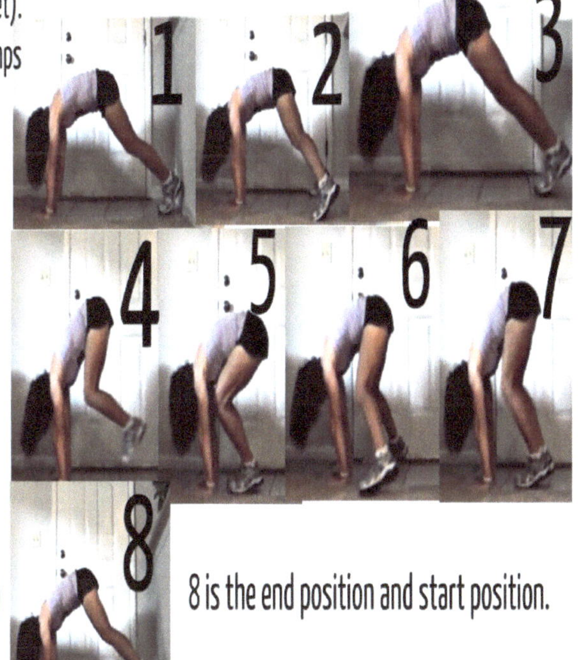

(BELOW) Advanced Hands Flat Triangular Plank Jack

Keep body tight in triangular position. Feet go out 2-3 feet and then land feet center flat together.

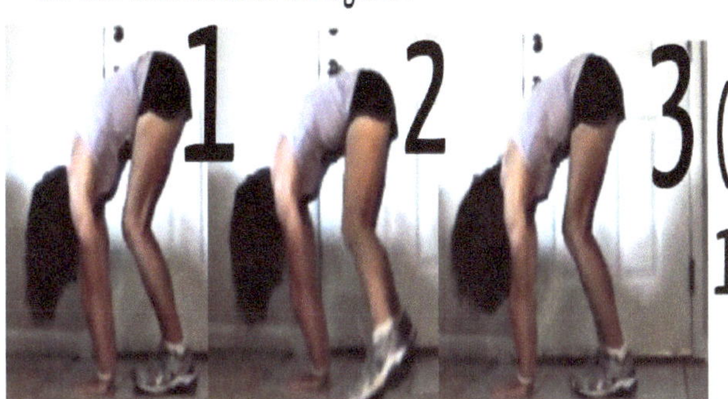

(L)

1+2+3 = 1 rep

8 is the end position and start position.

WRW Bone Density Builders AKA Aerobic Strength Planks (Plank Leap Series)

Goal: Develop strength, jumping height, and power off the feet.

Progressions: Complete in any order...modified or advanced depending on fitness level. Remember, Aquatic Aces only did Plank Leaps in shallow pool using wall (head out of water). You may do on land by kitchen counter. Alicia only does the advanced moves in training. Advanced start with just a few reps. Proper form is key. Modified go by time...Aquatic Aces would do only 1 set for 30 seconds to 2 minutes per exercise. NOTE: Arms are straight in all exercises.

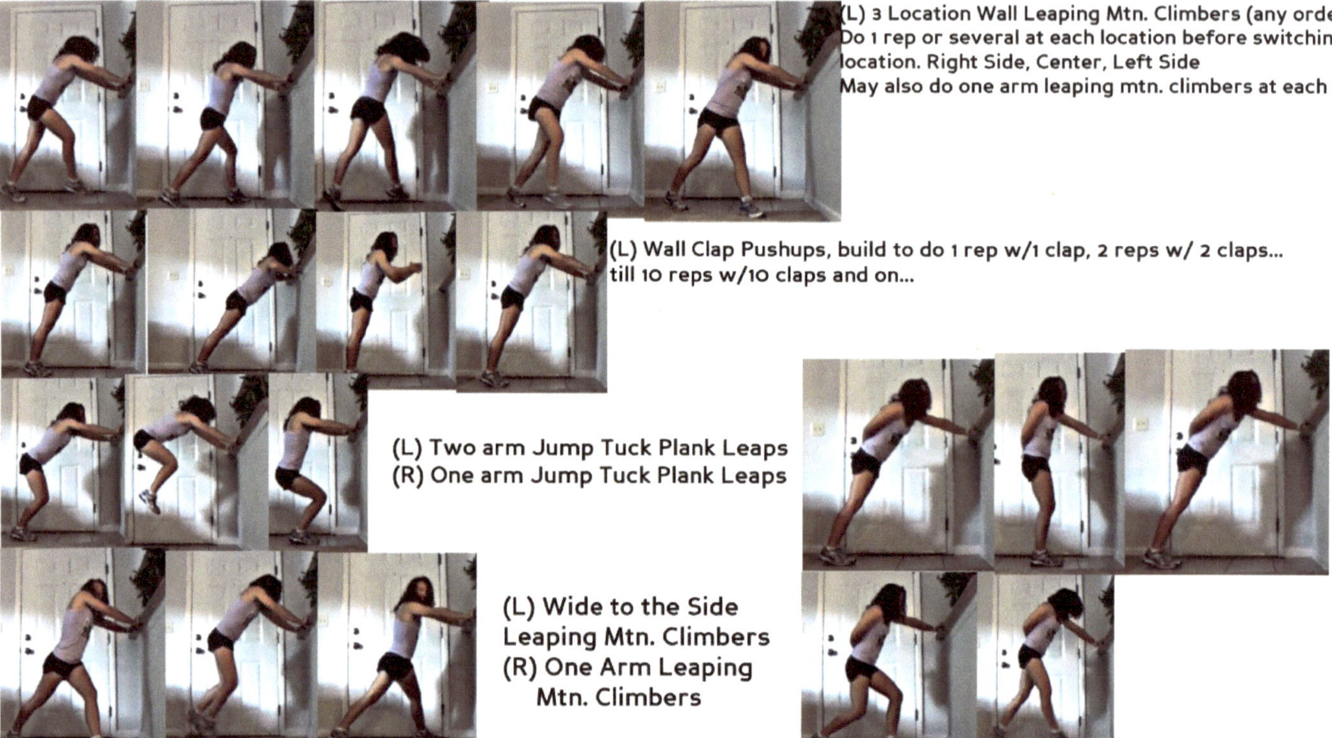

(L) 3 Location Wall Leaping Mtn. Climbers (any order)
Do 1 rep or several at each location before switching to next location. Right Side, Center, Left Side
May also do one arm leaping mtn. climbers at each location.

(L) Wall Clap Pushups, build to do 1 rep w/1 clap, 2 reps w/ 2 claps... till 10 reps w/10 claps and on...

(L) Two arm Jump Tuck Plank Leaps
(R) One arm Jump Tuck Plank Leaps

(L) Wide to the Side Leaping Mtn. Climbers
(R) One Arm Leaping Mtn. Climbers

Advanced Plank Leap Series

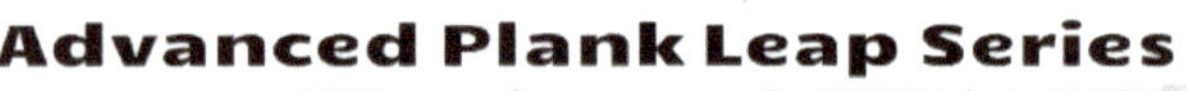

(L) Burpee Pushup with Over head clap and jump
This is a demo of one rep.

(L) One Arm Burpee Pushup with Over Head Clap and jump.
This is demo of one rep.

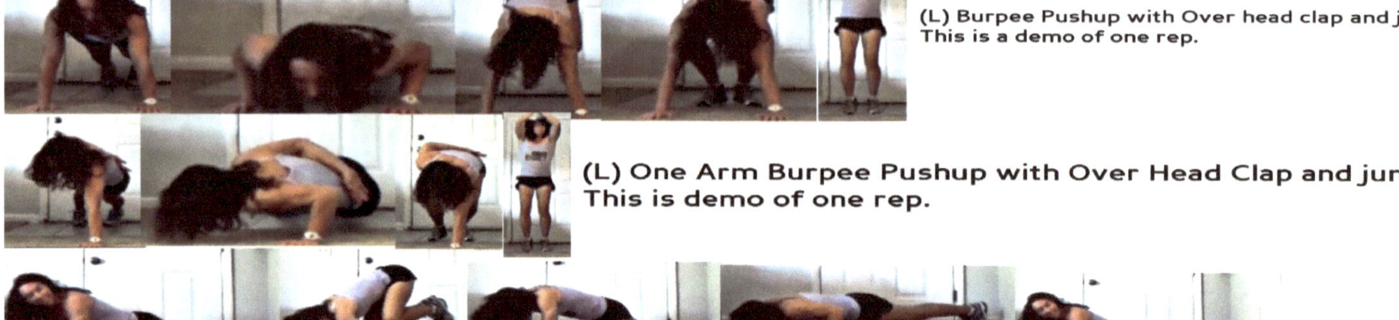

(ABOVE) High Knee Jump Tuck Pushup
Drive knees high in air to waist. Return to plank and pushup. This is one rep.

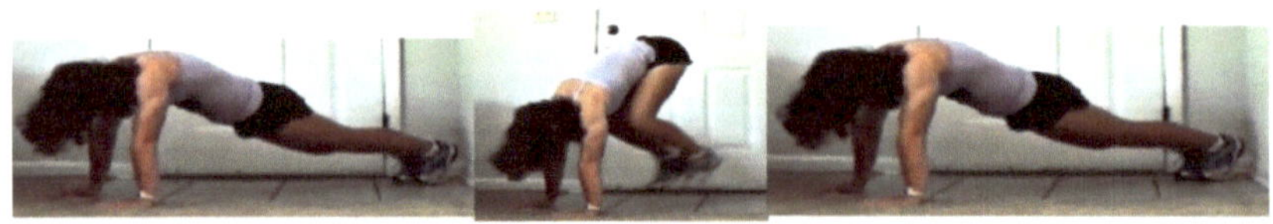

(L) High Knee Plank Jumps
Drive Knees to waist high in air and return to plank.

WRW Bone Density Builders AKA Aerobic Strength Planks (Plank Jump Series)

Goal: Develop power, strength, and jumping distance
Progressions: Complete in any order...modified or advanced depending on fitness level. Remember, Aquatic Aces only did
Plank Jumps in shallow water pool using wall (head out of water). You may do on land by kitchen counter. Alicia only does the
advanced moves in training. Advanced start with just a few reps. Proper form is key. Modified go by time...Aquatic Aces would
do only 1 set for 30 seconds to 2 minutes per exercise. NOTE: Arms are straight in all exercises except the Wall Wide to the Side.

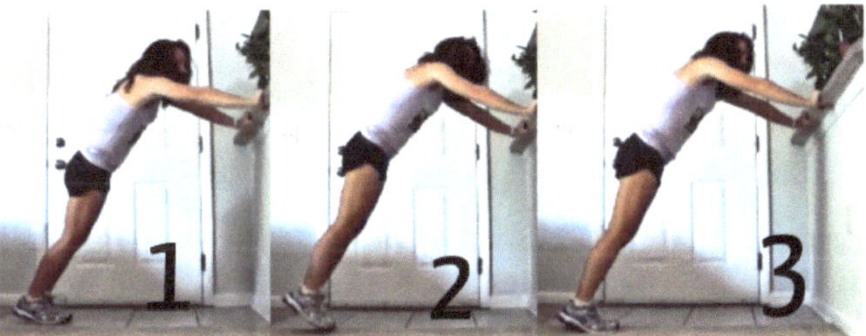

(ABOVE) Short Wall Speed Jumps side-to-side
Jumps are no more than hip -width apart.
Feet Stay togther. Stay diagonal.

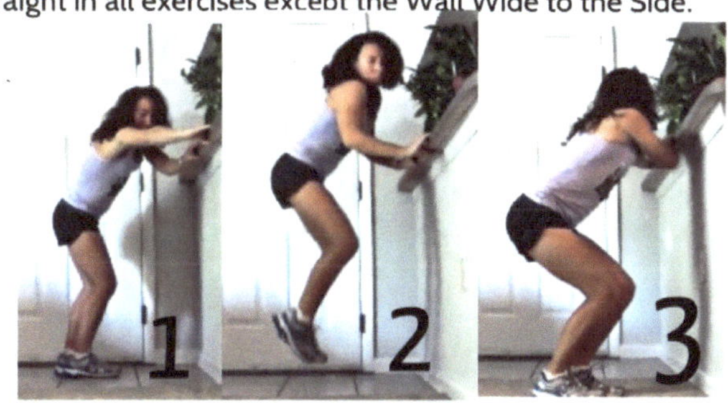

(ABOVE) Wall-Wide Side-to-Side... Keep feet together. Begin Jump with feet beyond the level of
the hand on whatever side you start. Take big jump to other side and land with feet beyond level of that hand.

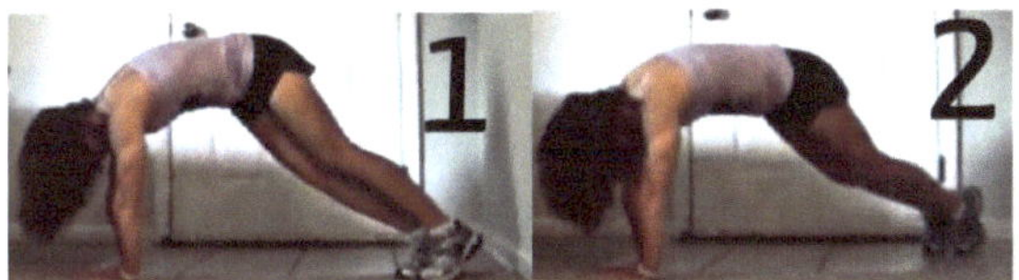

(ABOVE) Plank Jumps with feet moving
side-to-side in short space. Feet stay together.
It is like small bunny hops, while in plank.

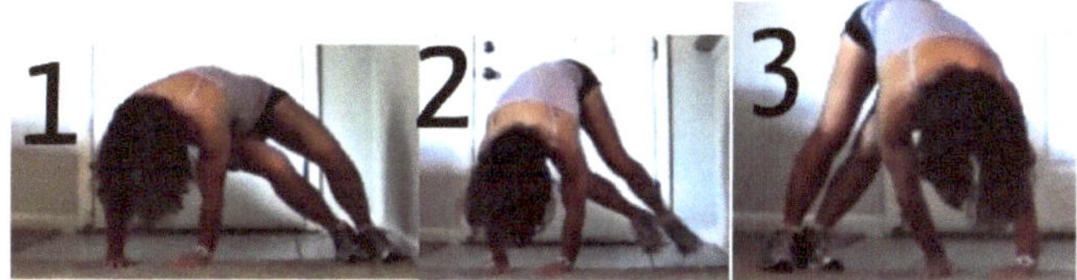

(ABOVE) Advanced Wide to the Side Plank Jumps
Begin with feet together and at level of one hand. Jump
big across body and land with feet together and at level
of other hand.

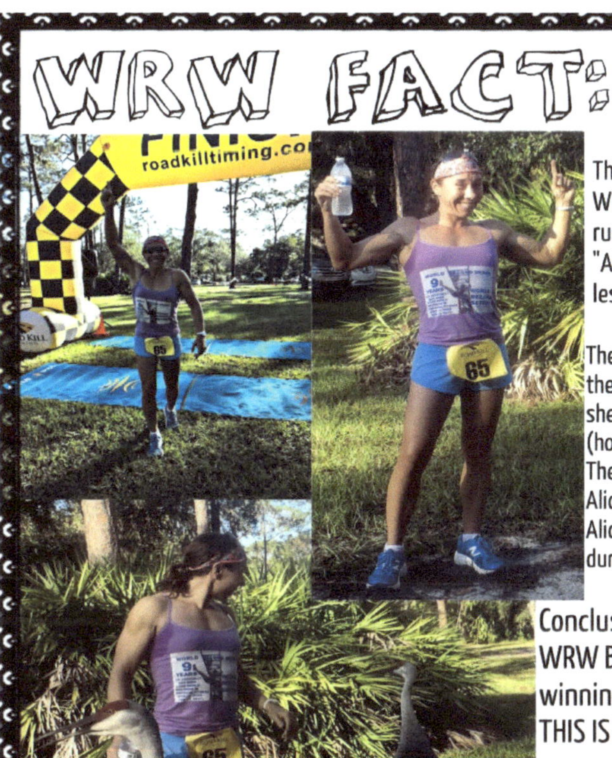

WRW FACT:

Alicia won the 2017 Run Childhood Cancer Out of Town
5k after 4-weeks of NEW "WRW Bone Density Building"
training program.

The "WRW Bone Density Building" Run Plan: Increase Frequency and duration of the
WRW Wellness Routines (two 30-60 minute sessions a week), while eliminating distance
running. Plan only allows completion of run interval training with floor only (advanced)
"Aerobic Strength Planks" 2-4 sessions a week. The total running mileage was 20 miles or
less each week for 4 weeks from Oct 9-Nov 5, 2017.

The Objective/Race Results: Goal is to see if new plan produces top results. Alicia would consider
the plan a success, if she was able to negative split, win, and even set a course record. Also,
she wanted to complete the event with a minimal level of perceived exertion
(how hard you feel like your body is working on scale 1-10). The lower the #, the better.
The Race Result: Alicia won first place overall out of men and women for her 118th career victory
Alicia also set the women's course record with her time of 21:04 on the sand trail at Moss Park.
Alicia finished the race with a perceived effort of 5 out of 10 and she was able to negative split
during the race... 6:55 at mile 1, 13:29 at mile 2 (6:34), and 21:04 at 5K. 6:48/AVG mile pace

Conclusion: The WRW Wellness Routines in combination with the
WRW Bone Density Builders greatly reduce training time and produce
winning results with minimal perceived exertion.
THIS IS DEFINITELY A KEEPER AND LONG-TERM WINNNG PROGRAM.

18

Thank you for reading WRW Wellness Routines and All the Best in Your Success

Alicia Weber officially set 1,000 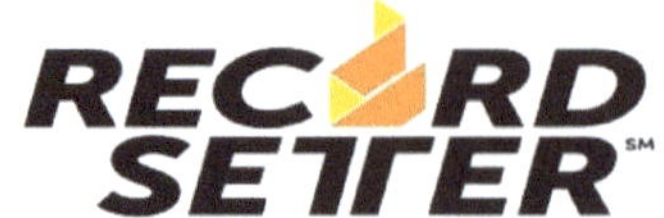 physical fitness records at Recordsetter World Records (www.recordsetter.com/user/AliciaWeber) from March 6, 2012 to January 23, 2017....1,000 records in 1,785 days (one record every 42 hours).

The LIST OF RECORDS is below. Key: CR = current record FR=former record OR=original record meaning Alicia created the record category. If a record only has one OR by it, then Alicia nor anyone else has re-set it and it is the current record. BR=someone broke the record Alicia held *=record is not counted in this time frame of March 6, 2012 –January 23, 2017

Record #	Description	Result/Date
1000	Most consecutive inverted row one-arm bean bag catch pull-ups	OR 11 pull-ups (1/23/17)
999-991	Most consecutive six-count plyometric plank jump sets in 2 minutes/7 sets, 3 minutes/10 sets, 4 minutes/13 sets, 5 minutes/15 sets, 6 minutes/18 sets, 7 minutes/21 sets, 8 minutes/25 minutes, 9 minutes/28 sets, and 10 minutes/32 sets	OR (1/23/17)
990	Most consecutive inverted row bean bag catch pull-ups	OR 7 pull-ups (1/23/17)
989	Fastest time to perform 100 consecutive side-center-side plank jumps	OR 2:47 min/sec (1/22/17)
988-975	Most consecutive side-center-side plank jumps in 15 minutes/402 jumps, 14 minutes/360 jumps, 13 minutes/330 jumps, 12 minutes/312 jumps, 11 minutes/282 jumps, 10 minutes/258 jumps, 9 minutes/228 jumps, 8 minutes/210 jumps, 7 minutes/174 jumps, 6 minutes/162 jumps, 5 minutes/144 jumps, 4 minutes/126 jumps, 3 minutes/108 jumps, and 2 minutes/72 jumps	OR (1/22/17)
974	Fastest Time to perform 100 consecutive V-Plank Jacks	OR 6:42.4 min/sec (1/22/17)
973-959	Most consecutive V-Plank Jacks in 15 mins/225 jacks, 14 mins/217 jacks, 13 mins/203 jacks, 12 mins/180 jacks, 11 mins/165 jacks, 10 mins/150 jacks, 9 mins/135 jacks, 8 mins/118 jacks, 7 mins/105 jacks, 6 mins/90 jacks, 5 mins/77 jacks, 4 mins/61 jacks, 3 mins/47 jacks, 2 mins/35 jacks, and one minute/25 jacks	OR (1/22/17)
958	Fastest Time to perform 100 consecutive volleyball sit-ups	OR 8:36.4 min/sec (1/22/17)
957-948	Most consecutive volleyball sit-ups (keeping volleyball in air) in 10 mins/117 sit-ups, 9 mins/104 sit-ups, 8 mins/90 sit-ups, 7 mins/78 sit-ups, 6 mins/64 sit-ups, 5 mins/50 sit-ups, 4 mins/40 sit-ups, 3 mins/33 sit-ups, 2 mins/25 sit-ups, and min/15 sit-ups	OR(1/22/17)
947-945	Fastest consecutive side-center-side plank jumps 200 jumps/7:50.57 min/sec, 300 jumps/11:43, 400 jumps/14:55.7	OR (1/22/17)
944	Most Consecutive Side-To-Side plank jumps in one minute	BR 42 Jumps (1/22/17)
943-942	Fastest time to perform 100 consecutive side-to-side plank jacks 3:41 min/sec OR, OR 200 plank jacks 9:26.77 min/sec	(1/21/17)
941-933	Most consecutive side-to-side plank jacks in 10 mins/216 jacks, 9 mins/190 jacks, 8 mins/170 jacks, 7 mins/150 jacks, 6 mins/130 jacks, 5 mins/120 jacks, 4 mins/105 jacks, 3 mins/80 jacks, 2 mins/57 jacks	OR (1/21/17)
932	Most straight leg raises in a minute doing a flexed bar hang (supinated grip)	OR 28 leg raises (1/20/17)
931	Most straight leg raises in a minute doing a flexed bar hang (pronated grip)	OR 27 leg raises (1/20/17)
930	Most consecutive pull-ups (with ascending ladder of knee-to-elbows (ie on second pull-up 2 reps of knee-to-elbows then 3rd with 3 reps etc.)	OR 9 pull-ups with 9 Knee-to-elbows (1/20/17)
929	Most consecutive chin-ups (with ascending ladder of knee-to-elbows ie on second chin-up 2 reps of knee-to-elbows then 3rd with 3 reps etc.)	OR 9 chin-ups with 9 knee-to-elbows (1/20/17)
928	Most consecutive staircase pull-ups (15 air steps per pull-up)	OR 10 pull-ups (1/20/17)
927	Fastest 100 yard one-foot hop on grass	OR 28.27 seconds (1/19/17)
926	Most Side-to-Side Plank Jumps in one minute	BR 36 jumps (1/19/17)
925-913	Most consecutive High Knee Jump Pushups in 6 mins/93 on (1/18/17) CR and 83 on (1/14/17) OR, 5 mins/84 on (1/18/17) CR and 75 on (1/14/17) OR, 4 mins/71 on (1/18/17) CR and 63 on (1/14/17) OR, 3 mins/60 on (1/18/17) CR and 55 on (1/14/17) OR, 2 mins/48 on (1/18/17) CR and 40 on (1/14/17) OR, one minute/34 on (1/18/17) CR and 31 on (1/14/17) OR	
912-911	Fastest time to perform 100 consecutive high knee jump pushups	6:31.37on (1/18/17) CR and OR 7:41.9 on (1/14/17)
910	Most consecutive moving chin-ups with ascending ladder knee-to-elbows (ie second chin-up has 2 knee-to-elbows, 3rd with 3 knee-to-elbows etc)	OR 10 chin-ups with 10 Knee-to-elbows (1/18/17)
909	Fastest time to perform 300 consecutive V-mountain climber exercises	OR 13:19.4 min/sec (1/14/17)

Record #	Description	Result/Date

908-894 Most Consecutive V-Mountain climber exercises in 15 mins/356 reps, 14 mins/320 reps, 13 mins/295 reps, 12 mins/270 reps, 11 mins/245 reps, 10 mins/225 reps, 9 mins/200 reps, 8 mins/175 reps, 7 mins/150 reps, 6 mins/130 reps, *5 mins/171 reps(10/6/17) CR and 116 reps (1/14/17) OR ,*4 mins/140 reps (10/6/17) CR and 90 reps (1/14/17) OR, *3 mins/110 reps (10/6/17) CR and 70 reps (1/14/17) OR, *2 mins/85 reps (10/6/17) CR and 55 reps (1/14/17) OR, and *minute/62 reps (10/6/17) CR and 36 reps (1/14/17) OR

893   Fastest time to perform 100 consecutive V-mountain climber exercises   OR 4:15 min/sec   (1/14/17)

892   Fastest Combined 100 yard right leg and 100 yard left leg hop (both legs hopped in 28.27 seconds)   OR   56.54 seconds (11/14/17)

891-883 Most consecutive high knee jump pushups in *15 mins/182 reps (12/5/17) CR and 165 reps (1/14/17) OR, 14 mins/150 reps (1/14/17) CR, *13 mins/157 (12/5/17) CR and 142 reps (1/14/17) OR, 12 mins/135 reps (1/14/17) OR, 11 mins/131 reps (1/14/17) OR, 10 mins/126 reps (1/14/17) OR, 9 mins/113 reps (1/14/17) OR, 8 mins/105 reps (1/14/17) OR, 7 mins/92 reps (1/14/17) OR

882-881 Most consecutive moving staircase pull-ups (move on monkey bar with each pull-up rep and do 15 air steps per pull-up)
CR 11 pull-ups (1/13/17) and OR 10 pull-ups (1/12/17)

880   Most consecutive moving 10lbs weighted (total weight of ankle weights) staircase pull-ups (move on monkey bar with each pull-up and do 15 air steps)   OR   6 pull-ups (1/12/17)

879-875 Most hands-flat triangle star squat in 5 mins/206 reps, 4 mins/165 reps, 3 mins/122 reps, 2 mins/85 reps, min/68 reps OR (1/11/17)

874-864 Most consecutive strict chest-touching-ground reptile-pushups in 10 mins/186 reps CR (1/10/17), 10 mins/126 reps OR (9/1/14), 9 mins/164 reps CR (1/10/17), 8 mins/154 reps CR (1/10/17), 7 mins/139 reps CR (1/10/17), 6 mins/127 reps CR (1/10/17), 5 mins/114 reps CR (1/10/17), 4 mins/103 reps CR (1/10/17), 4 mins/101 reps FR (9/26/14), 4 mins/62 reps OR (9/1/14)

863   Longest one-arm archer flexed bar hang   OR 53.28 seconds   (1/10/17)

862-860 Most 2 armed & 1 -legged leaping mountain climber in 5 minutes 228 reps CR (1/8/17), 203 reps FR (1/2/17), 160 reps OR (7/30/12)

859-855 Fastest time to perform Tiger bend pushups, while throwing bean bag and drawing V's with legs 50 reps/4:27.57 min/sec, 40 reps/3:53.13 min/sec, 30 reps/3:11.37 min/sec, 20 reps/2:13.1 min/sec, 10 reps/55.2 seconds   OR   (1/7/17)

854-850 Fastest time to perform one arm gliding disc mountain climbers, while throwing and catching a bean bag a certain number of times 50 catches/1:38.30 min/sec, 40 catches/1:20.5 min/sec, 30 catches/1:02 min/sec, 20 catches/40.8 seconds, 10 catches/16.23 seconds
OR   (1/7/17)

849-842 Fastest consecutive plank holds, while throwing and catching a bean bag a certain number of times 95 catches/1:45.6 min/sec, 85 catches/1:34.43 min/sec, 75 catches/1:21.27 min/sec, 65 catches/1:06.3 min/sec, 55 catches/53.67 seconds, 35 catches/38.42 seconds, 25 catches/18.6 seconds, 15 catches/10.63 seconds   OR   (1/7/17)

841-837 Fastest time to perform bean bag catches, while doing a certain number of consecutive jump tuck pushups 10 pushups/25.20 seconds, 20 pushups/1:38.50 min/sec, 30 pushups/2:36.7 min/sec, 40 pushups/3:27.97 min/sec, 50 pushups/4:28.0 min/sec OR   (1/7/17)

837-835 Fastest time to perform gliding plank jacks, while throwing and catching a bean bag a certain number of times 15 catches/23.29 seconds, 10 catches/13.50 seconds, 5 catches/6.27 seconds   OR   (1/7/17)

834-833 Fastest time to perform one arm gliding plank jacks with a certain number of bean bag throws and catches 25 catches/1:16.57 min/sec, 20 catches/1:01.30 min/sec   OR   (1/7/17)

832-828 Fastest time to hold a crabwalk position and throw and catch a bean bag overhead (without dropping it) 50 catches/ 48.37 seconds, 40 catches/38.07 seconds, 30 catches/28.5 seconds, 20 catches/18 seconds, 10 catches/8 seconds   OR   (1/7/17)

827-824 Most Consecutive Pushups in Three Minutes *167 reps (10/18/17) CR, 162 reps (1/20/17) FR, 160 reps (12/27/16) FR, 159 reps (11/17/16) FR, and OR 156 reps (11/1/16)

823   Longest L-Sit Hold on a Bar   BR   45.4 seconds (8/29/16)

822-821   Fastest time to perform 100 tennis ball wall bounces with 100 pushups *6:12.57 min/sec (5/9/17) CR, 6:26.3 min/sec (9/22/16) FR, 7:03.11 (4/24/14) OR

820   Fastest time to perform 10 one-arm Tiger Bend Pushups *25.5 seconds (12/31/17) CR, OR 26.7 seconds (11/26/16)

819-816   Most Consecutive Bar L-Dips *52 reps (12/11/17) CR, 49 reps (12/21/16) FR, 48 reps (9/21/16) FR, 45 reps (5/26/16) FR, OR 41 reps (5/6/16)

815 Fastest time to perform 100 consecutive alternating forearm-to-tricep extension pushups *6:19.33 (8/9/17) CR, OR 7:47.10 (1/1/17)

814-812 Most hanging Swiss Ball Ab rolls in 3 minutes/25 rolls, 2 minutes/18 rolls, 1 minute/12 rolls   OR   (1/6/17)

811-804   Most 2-armed and 1-legged leaping mtn. climber in 4 minutes/ 204 reps (1/4/17) CR, 4 mins/151 reps (1/2/17) OR, 3 mins/168 reps (1/4/17) CR, 3 mins/121 reps (1/2/17) OR, 2 mins/124 reps (1/4/17) CR, 2 mins/86 reps (1/2/17) OR, min/78 reps (1/4/17) CR, OR min/61 reps (1/2/17)

803-802   Most consecutive archer-pushups in 3 minutes 63 (12/30/16) CR, OR 53 (12/20/16)

801-799 Fastest time to complete 100 strict one-arm squat thrusts 2:17.63 (12/30/16) CR, 3:19.77 (10/5/15) FR, OR 5:55.33 (9/1/14)

798-797 Most extreme one arm exercise reps in 2 mins (first minute one arm reptile pushups then minute of one arm squat thrusts) 56 reps (12/30/16) CR, OR 40 reps (9/1/14)

Record #	Description	Result/Date

Record # — **Description** — **Result/Date**

796 — Most consecutive spiderman pushups in 25 minutes — OR 435 reps (12/129/16)

795--792 — Most consecutive reps completed in "Triple Tree Pull-Up" Challenge (Max L-Pullups, L-scissor Pull-Ups, Pull-ups) 38 reps (12/26/16) CR, 36 reps (12/25/16) FR, 35 reps (12/23/16) FR, 30 reps (11/26/16) OR

791 — Most consecutive L-Chin-Ups on a tree branch in one minute — OR 25 reps (12/26/16)

790-787 — Most consecutive L-Pull-Ups on a Tree branch in minute — 27 (12/24/16) CR, 24 (12/23/16) FR, 22 (11/27/16) FR, OR 20 (11/26/16)

786-782 — Most stretched out pushups in one minute — 49 (12/23/16) CR, 46 (10/22/13) FR, 44 (9/5/13) FR, 39 (3/29/13) FR, OR 25 (8/13/12)

781-780 — Most sumo squat arm flaps in Three Minutes — 107 reps (12/23/16) CR, OR 103 reps (11/28/16)

779-778 — Fastest time to perform 150 consecutive reptile-pushups — 7:00.53 min/sec (12/22/16) CR, OR 7:23.23 min/sec (12/15/16)

777 — Fastest time to perform 125 consecutive reptile-pushups — OR 5:47.53 min/sec (12/22/16)

776-775 — Most consecutive thick bar L-chin ups — 29 reps (12/19/16) CR, OR 24 reps (12/8/16)

774-773 — Most consecutive thick bar L pull-ups — 29 reps (12/19/16) CR, OR 25 reps (12/8/16)

772 — Farthest L-Sit Incline Parallel Arm Walk in One Minute — OR 10 feet (12/8/16)

771-765 — Most Full Rep Towel L Pull-Ups 45 reps (12/8/16) CR, 41 reps (12/17/13) FR, 40 reps (6/19/13) FR, 35 reps (4/3/13 FR), 30 reps (11/6/12) FR, 27 reps (8/16/12) FR, FR 22 reps (6/17/12)

764-762 Longest Pike Hold Hanging from Men's Gymnastics Still Rings 73.40 secs(12/1/16)CR, 72.51 secs(8/29/15) FR, FR 61.9 sec(4/16/15)

761-760 Fastest mile cross country run with 100 consecutive pushups at the end 7:55.7 min/sec (10/20/16) CR, OR 8:00.4 min/sec (6/29/16)

759-752 Most consecutive strict chin-ups on thick bar 59 (12/20/16) CR, 56 (11/8/16) FR, 53 (11/13/16) FR, 48 (9/21/16) FR, 46 (6/8/16) FR, 41 (5/28/16) FR, 39 (5/26/16) FR, OR 37 (5/8/16)

751 — Most consecutive gymnastic ring archer pull-ups in one minute — OR 12 reps (11/29/16)

750 — Most consecutive gymnastic ring archer chin-ups in one minute — OR 11 reps (11/29/16)

749-746 — Longest time hanging from a tree branch — 3:33.73 (11/26/16) CR, 3:03.59 (5/18/15)FR, 2:39.52 (8/28/14)FR, FR 2:13.40 (12/25/13)

745-739 Most Full Rep Towel Pull-Ups 53 (11/6/16)CR, All FRs 52 (6/28/16), 47 (6/4/13), 45 (8/31/12), 40 (6/22/12), 37 (5/27/12), 35 (3/18/12)

738-734 Most Consecutive Spiderman Pushups in Minute 64 (11/18/16) CR, 54 (9/7/16) FR, 52 (12/29/15) FR, 45 (11/7/15) FR, OR 35 (11/2/15)

733 Most points scored in a 900 round barebow archery shoot @ 20 yds for 3x(30 arrows + min of archer pushups) 622 Points OR (11/5/16)

732-730 — Most consecutive strict pull-ups on thick bar — 59 (11/8/16) CR, 58 (6/3/16) FR, OR 54 (5/6/16)

729-723 Most Half-Rep Towel Pull-Ups 72 (11/6/16) CR, All FRs 71 (6/28/16), 64(6/19/13), 56 (4/3/13), 54 (8/31/16), 49(6/24/12), 42 (5/27/12)

722-717 Most strict moving monkey bar pull-ups 36 (11/14/16)CR, 35(9/24/15)FR, 30(1/5/15)FR, 26(12/24/14)FR, 23(9/25/14)FR,OR 21(9/19/14)

716 — Farthest Flexed Hang Bar Arm Walk in One Minute — *97ft (8/25/17) CR, OR 90ft (7/28/13)

715 — Most Consecutive Sprinter Sit-Ups — *410 reps (8/12/17) CR, OR 305 reps (10/20/14)

714-707 Most push-ups on 3 medicine balls in 2 minutes *84 reps (7/30/17) CR, OR 80 reps (7/4/16) 3 minutes *111 reps (7/29/17) CR, 102 reps (7/4/16) FR, 85 reps (3/28/15) FR, OR 74 reps (8/21/14) 4 minutes *131 reps (7/29/17) CR, OR 115 reps (7/4/16) 5 minutes *152 reps (7/29/17) CR, OR 132 reps (7/4/16) one minute *61 reps (7/27/17) CR, 60 reps (7/5/16) FR, 57 reps (7/4/16) FR, *OR 52 reps (2/7/12)

706-704 — Most consecutive pushups with an elevated leg on 3 medicine balls in one minute *51 reps (7/29/17) CR, 46 reps (3/28/15) FR, 41 reps (10/30/12) FR, OR 39 reps (4/5/12)

703 — Fastest time to complete 100 hanging leg L raises — *2:19.33 min/sec (5/24/17) CR, OR 2:26.87 min/sec (7/18/16)

702-700 Fastest time to complete 250 perfect pull-ups and 250 perfect reptile pushups *21:00.17 min/sec (5/14/17) CR, 22:58.53 (2/10/15) FR, 30:48 (6/25/13) FR, OR 41:50 (11/17/12)

699 — Fastest time to complete 300 thick grip pull-ups and one mile cross country — *23:50.8 (3/17/17) CR, OR 30:46.7 (5/19/16)

698-697 — Most Pull-Ups in 3 minutes — BR 103 reps (6/17/16), OR 101 reps (9/27/15)

696 — Most double burpee pushups in one minute — BR 23 reps (10/26/15)

695-694 — Most consecutive ipsilateral one arm one leg pushups — BR 12 reps (8/1/15), BR 7 reps (7/13/15)

693-691 — Most knuckle pushups in one minute — BR 97 reps (6/16/15), BR 85 reps (7/22/14), BR 69 reps (6/2/14)

690 — Most consecutive 4-finger pushups (female only category) — BR 22 reps (4/20/15)

689-688 — Most consecutive one arm one legged push-ups — BR 47 reps (4/6/15), BR 21 reps (3/6/15)

687 — Most consecutive jump squats in 30 seconds — BR 37 reps (2/3/15)

686-683 Fastest to do 100 side-to-side V-Squats All BRs 47.5 secs(10/17/14), 66.52 secs(8/21/14), 76 secs(12/17/13), OR 82.3 secs (11/27/13)

682-680 — Most sit-ups in One Minute — All BRs 72 reps (7/24/14), 62 reps (1/1/13), 59 reps (4/12/12), *55 reps (2/21/12)

679-678 — Most one-armed burpee exercises in 2 minutes, while wearing a Boxing Glove — BR 54 reps (11/7/12), BR 46 reps (11/2/12)

677 — Most consecutive flying superman push-ups — BR 40 reps 5/27/12, *BR 31 reps (2/28/12)

676 — Most deep squats in 3 minutes with arms held out — BR 167 reps (3/29/12)

675-665 Most consecutive knee tucks *1,157 reps(9/6/17) CR, 1, 140 reps (11/4/15) FR, 714 reps ((10/3/15) FR, 675 reps (6/30/14) FR, 668 reps (10/1/13) FR, 648 reps (7/20/13) FR, 513 reps (12/6/12) FR, 446 reps (8/13/12) FR, 402 reps (6/9/12) FR, 310 reps (5/24/12) FR, 254 reps (4/27/12) FR, *FR 138 reps (2/27/12)

664   Most one leg burpee pushups in 2 minutes using alternating legs   BR 34 reps (8/6/12)

663-662 Most pushups on 3 medicine balls in a minute (female only category) *61 reps (7/27/17) CR, 60 reps (7/5/16) FR, 57 reps (7/4/16) FR, *OR 52 reps (2/7/12)

661-660 Most flutter presses in 5 minutes using 40% of one's body weight   113 reps (8/6/14) CR, OR 105 reps (8/13/12)

659-657 Most consecutive plyometric clap pull-ups   32 reps (10/17/16) CR, 28 reps (7/31/15) FR, OR 25 reps (4/5/15)

656-654 Most situps on a floating paddleboard in 2 minutes   81 sit-ups (10/15/16) CR, 56 sit-ups (9/26/15) FR, FR 51 sit-ups (12/14/13)

653   Most pushups on a floating paddleboard in 90 seconds   CR 63 push-ups (10/15/16)

652-647 Most consecutive double bar flexed hang knee tucks 159 reps (10/13/16) CR, 142 (1/12/15) FR, 139 (9/5/13) FR, 125 (4/3/13) FR, 100 7/22/12) FR, OR 82 reps (7/11/12)

646   Most reps doing "Hurricane Matthew" Arm-Ab Fitness Challenge in 30 minutes   CR 312 reps (10/7/16)

645-644 Greatest distance climbed in Monkey Bar L-Sit Climb in 30 seconds   CR 48ft (10/6/16), OR 36ft (6/9/16)

643-635 Greatest distance to arm walk and foot glide in 5 minutes CR 175 yds (9/25/16), OR 165 yds (6/18/16) In 4 minutes OR 140 yds (9/25/16), In 3 minutes CR 115 yds(9/25/16) and OR 110 yds (6/18/16) In 2 minutes CR 90 yds (9/25/16) and OR 80 yds (6/18/16), In a minute CR 55 yds (9/25/16) and OR 45 yds (6/18/16)

634-629 Most pull-ups in one minute followed by most chin-ups in one minute (max 6 mins rest btw exercises) 56/55 reps (9/24/16) CR, 55/51 reps (8/29/15) FR, 50/46 reps (6/9/15) FR, 47/42 reps (6/2/14) FR, 43/40 reps (2/8/14) FR, OR 41/39 reps (3/27/13)

628-625 Most consecutive spiderman push-ups in 2 minutes 79 reps (9/7/16) CR, 77 (12/29/15) FR, 66 (11/7/15) FR, OR 56 reps (11/2/15)

624-622 Most consecutive spiderman push-ups in 3 minutes 101 reps (9/7/16) CR, 97 (12/29/15) FR, 87 (11/7/15) FR, OR 77 reps (11/2/15)

621-618 Most consecutive spiderman push-ups in 4 minutes 120 reps (9/7/16) CR, 115 (12/29/15) FR, 105 (11/7/15) FR, OR 100 reps (11/2/15)

617-614 Most consecutive spiderman push-ups in 5 minutes 140 reps (9/7/16) CR, 135 (12/29/15) FR, 125 (11/7/15) FR, OR 119 reps (11/2/15)

613-611 Most consecutive decline locked-finger push-ups in 5 minutes 92 reps (9/5/16) CR, 85 (5/24/16) FR, OR 77 reps (5/9/16)

610-607 Fastest time to complete 100 strict pull-ups and 100 burpee push-ups with end jump and overhead clap 10:07.60 min/sec (9/3/16) CR, 10:22.66 min/sec (11/25/14) FR, 11:55.48 min/sec (9/16/12) FR, OR 12:42.96 min/sec (8/15/12)

606-605   Most consecutive L-Pull-ups in one minute   28 pull-ups (9/2/16) CR, OR 26 pull-ups (7/16/16)

604   Fastest 100 meter grass Ab Wheel walk   OR 4:17 min/sec (8/20/16)

603 Most consecutive increasing bar dip holds (must hold at bottom of dip and top in # of seconds of the rep ie 16 reps=16 seconds) OR 16 dips (8/16/16)

602-601   Most consecutive flexed bar hang bent knee to elbow exercises (pronated grip)   80 reps (8/14/16) CR, OR 75 reps (7/11/15)

600-595   Most strict concrete knuckle squat thrusts in one minute 87 (8/13/16) CR, 70 (12/31/15) FR, 65 (10/24/15) FR, 61 (1/11/15) FR, 56 (12/24/14) FR, FR 46 (9/1/14)

594-590 Most consecutive straight arm and leg bar hanging L-Lifts 21 lifts (8/7/16) CR, 18 (7/28/16) FR, 16 (12/19/13) FR, 15 (3/29/13) FR, OR 10 lifts (8/13/12)

589 Most non-stop combos of leg lifts and straight leg holds on the floor 2,030 leg lifts and a total of 34 minutes of holds (7/30/16) CR, *OR 1,500 leg lifts and a total of 25 minutes of holds (3/11/11)

588-586 Longest swiss ball leg lifts cadence test (20 leg lifts per min till failure) 31 minutes (7/20/16) CR, 19 minutes (12/13/12) FR, OR 10 minutes (11/11/12)

585-584 Most hollow body rocks, while balancing turtle on stomach   20 reps (7/10/16) CR, OR 11 reps (11/28/13)

583   Most strict pull-ups in one hour (using a straight bar)   OR 1,070 pull-ups (6/22/16)

582-581 Most strict pull-ups in 30 minutes (using a straight bar)   595 reps (6/22/16) CR, OR 575 reps (9/27/15)

580-577 Most strict chest-touching-ground reptile-pushups in 2 minutes   71 (6/21/16) CR, 68 (9/27/14) FR, 63 (9/26/14) FR, OR 36 (9/1/14)

576-573 Farthest arm walk and foot glide in 15 minutes OR 400 yards (6/18/16), In 20 minutes OR 550 yards (6/18/16), In 10 minutes 200 yards (6/18/16) CR, OR 240 yards (6/13/16)

572-568 Most reps completed in 3 minutes of strict pull-ups and 3 minutes of headstand presses 120 reps (6/17/16) CR, 105 (6/3/15) FR, 100 (12/16/13) FR, 90 (7/24/12) FR, OR 88 reps (5/18/12)

567-565 Most 90 degree flexed bar hang knee-to-elbow raises in 30 minutes 620 reps (6/10/16) CR, 475 reps (7/3/14) FR, OR 374 (1/17/13)

564   Fastest 2 mile cross country run with 200 consecutive pushups at the end   OR 18:41.4 min/sec (6/8/16)

563-561 Most consecutive decline locked-finger pushups in 15 minutes OR 205 (6/3/16), In 10 minutes 145 (6/3/16) CR, OR 138 (5/24/16)

560   Most Florida runners participating in one mile cross country race for Global Running Day   OR 6 runners (6/1/16)

559-552 Most decline locked-finger pushups in 4 minutes 75 (5/24/16) CR, OR 63 (5/9/16) In 3 minutes 60 (5/24/16) CR, OR 50 (5/9/16) In 2 minutes 45 (5/24/16) CR, OR 35 (5/9/16) In one minute 30 (5/24/16) CR, OR 25 (5/9/16)

551-550   Most consecutive L-Sit False Grip Chin-Ups   20 (5/7/16) CR, FR 16 (1/19/15)

549   Most consecutive back-of-hand pushups in 15 minutes   OR 212 reps (5/3/16)

548-543   Most consecutive archer dips   25 (4/23/16) CR, 23 (4/5/16) FR, 21 (1/31/16) FR, 19 (1/14/16) FR, 16 (12/20/15) FR, OR 12 (12/18/15)

542-541   Fastest 300 reps with strict form (100 pushups, 100 dips, 100 pull-ups)   10:20.5 min/sec (4/14/16) CR, OR 10:47.57 (2/24/16)

540   Most consecutive flexed hang hammer grip bent knee-to-elbow exercise   OR 84 reps (4/3/16)

539-538   Fastest time for 1,000 consecutive chest-touching-ground pushups   46:26 min/sec (3/20/16) CR, OR 46:49.5 min/sec (7/4/14)

537-527   Most Shoulder-level perfect pull-ups 62 (3/12/16) CR, 61 (3/9/15) FR, 57 (2/6/14) FR, 55 (1/14/14) FR, 54 (9/8/13) FR, 53 (8/23/13) FR, 41 (6/19/13) FR, 35 (5/20/13) FR, 33 (3/12/13) FR, OR 31 (12/16/12)

526 Fastest 600 rep upper body challenge (100 strict pull-ups, 100 consecutive reptile-pushups, 100 chin-ups, 100 consecutive pushups, 100 bar dips with another strict 100 pull-ups)   OR 32:38.87 min/sec (2/21/16)

525-523 Longest TRX knee tuck pushup cadence test (20 knee tuck pushups per minute till failure) 16 mins (2/5/16) CR, 10 mins (1/22/14) FR, OR 5 mins (8/29/12)

522-514 Most close grip inverted rows 113 (2/3/16) CR, 107 (1/31/16) FR, 90 (1/13/16) FR, 80 (9/22/15) FR, 70 (4/1/15) FR, 66 (1/8/15) FR, 61 (9/11/14) FR, 56 (12/12/13) FR, 51 (7/6/12) FR

513-511   Most plyometric inverted row chin-ups   74 (1/31/16) CR, 65 (10/28/15) FR, FR 45 (9/25/14)

510-507 Most plyometric inverted rows (pull-ups)   71 (1/31/16) CR, 63 (10/28/15) FR, 52 (9/25/14) FR, FR 41 (7/20/12)

506-504   Fastest time to do 5 variation 400-rep consecutive pushups   19:38.57 (1/17/16) CR, 21:53.29 (5/10/14) FR,OR 29:27.63 (6/1/13)

503-497 Most consecutive inverted row pull-ups 118 reps (1/17/16) CR, 105 reps (9/24/15) FR, 82 reps (1/5/15) FR, 70 reps (8/3/14) FR, 56 reps (9/5/13) FR, 52 reps (4/3/13) FR, FR 48 reps (7/15/12)

496-490 Most consecutive inverted rows 111 (1/14/16) CR, 105 (9/23/15) FR, 90 (1/5/15) FR, 71 (8/3/14) FR, 63 (9/5/13) FR, 62 (3/30/13) FR, OR 58 (7/16/12)

489-485 Most strict concrete knuckle squat thrusts in 3 mins/150 reps (12/31/15) CR, 146 reps (10/24/15)FR, 130 reps (1/11/15)FR, 126 reps (12/24/14) FR, OR 110 reps (9/1/14)

484-481   Most deep squats in 7 minutes 341, In 8 minutes 376, in 9 minutes 420, in 10 minutes 464 All ORs on (12/31/15)

480-476 Most strict concrete knuckle squat thrusts in 2 mins/109 reps (12/31/15) CR, 104 reps (10/24/15) FR, 96 reps (1/11/15) FR, 92 reps (12/24/14) FR, OR 75 reps (9/1/14)

475-469 Most consecutive spiderman pushups in 30 minutes 511 reps (12/29/15), 20 mins 375 reps (12/29/15) both OR, in 10 minutes 235 reps (12/29/15) CR, 225 (11/7/15) FR, OR 212 reps (11/2/15) In 15 minutes 325 reps (12/29/15) CR, OR 316 reps (11/7/15)

468-466 Most strict chest-touching-ground one arm push-ups in 2 minutes 37 reps (12/25/15) CR, 33 reps (8/16/14) FR, OR 30 reps (7/11/14)

465-462 Most consecutive strict one-armed pushups in 2 minutes (arm just bends to 90 degrees) 96 reps (12/25/15) CR, 93 reps (8/16/14) FR, 92 reps (5/29/14) FR, OR 79 reps (2/21/13)

461-456 Most strict one arm chest-touching-ground reptile-pushups in 3 minutes 38 reps (12/23/15) CR, 34 reps (10/13/15) FR, 30 reps (4/1/15) FR, 26 reps (12/31/14) FR, 22 reps (9/25/14) FR, OR 16 reps (9/1/14)

455-451 Most strict one arm chest-touching-ground reptile pushups in one minute 20 reps (12/23/15) CR, 17 reps (10/13/15) FR, 15 reps (12/31/14) FR, 12 reps (9/25/14) FR, OR 10 reps (9/1/14)

450-439 Most consecutive one-arm balance T-elevated Leg Pushups in certain time frames: 5 mins/75 reps (12/19/15) CR, 54 reps (12/12/15 OR, 4 mins/60 reps (12/19/15) CR, 42 reps (12/12/15) OR, 3 mins/45 reps (12/19/15) CR, 31 reps (12/12/15) OR, 2 mins/33 reps (12/19/15) CR, 22 reps (12/12/15) OR, 1 min/18 reps (12/19/15) CR, 15 reps (12/12/15) OR, 15 mins/153 reps (12/12/15) OR, OR 10 mins/103 reps (12/12/15)

438-433 Most consecutive bar dips in 5 minutes (arms breaking 90 degrees and then going into extension) 133 reps (11/20/15) CR, 127 reps (8/6/15) FR, 103 reps (11/13/14) FR, 95 reps (7/29/14) FR, 91 reps (5/3/12) FR, OR 85 reps (4/4/12)

432   Fastest 100 consecutive bar dips (arms breaking 90 degrees then going to extension)   OR   2:59.2 min/sec (11/20/15)

431-421   Most opposite arm and leg leaping mountain climber exercises in certain time frames: 5 mins/175 reps (11/18/15) CR, 115 reps (11/13/12) FR, 95 reps (7/30/12) OR, 4 mins/131 reps (11/18/15) CR, 81 reps (11/17/15) OR, 3 mins/91 reps (11/18/15) CR, 70 reps (11/17/15) OR, 2 mins/70 reps (11/18/15) CR, 50 reps (11/17/15) OR, OR 1 min/42 reps (11/18/15)

420-419 Fastest 100 leaping mtn. climber and 100 chest-touching-ground locked finger pushups   4:31.5 min/sec(11/17/15) CR, OR 5:56.8 min/sec (8/19/14)

418-414 Most straight leg curl-ups with 10lbs medicine ball in 3 minutes 218 reps (11/17/15) CR, 215 reps (4/3/13) FR, 203 reps (11/2/12) FR, 135 reps (8/6/12) FR, OR 80 reps (8/13/12)

413-407 Most consecutive elevated leg balance T-pushups in one minute/ 20 reps (11/8/15) OR, 2 mins/35 reps (11/8/15) OR, 3 mins/50 (11/8/15) OR, 4 mins/60 reps (11/8/15) OR, 5 mins/74 reps (11/8/15) OR, 10 mins/140 reps (11/8/15) OR, OR 15 mins/202 reps (11/8/15)   23

<u>**Record #**</u>   **Description**   **Result/Date**

406-404 Most strict chest-touching-ground reptile pushups in 3 minutes 93 reps (11/1/15) CR, 84 reps (9/26/14) FR, OR 50 reps (9/1/14)

403-399 Fastest 100 chest-touching-ground reptile pushups (in minutes/seconds) 3:14.23 (11/1/15)CR, 3:28.98 (7/30/15) FR, 3:29.4 (4/1/15) FR, 3:55 (9/26/14) FR, OR 7:48.82 (9/1/14)

398   Fastest 400-meter dash with 10 yard archery bullseye   OR 1:20.31 (min/sec) 10/26/15

397   Longest 90 degree static hold push-up with a 25lbs weight on back   CR 1:01.6 (min/sec) 10/26/15

396-393 Farthest distance arm walked on monkey bars in minute 190ft (10/17/15) CR, 120ft (9/26/13) BR, 108ft (9/3/13) FR, OR 100ft(7/28/13)

392-391   Most consecutive 3 finger one arm inverted row pull-ups   25 reps (10/15/15) CR, OR 15 reps (3/30/15)

390-387 Most inverted rows using 2 fingers on each hand   48 reps (10/15/15) CR, 45 (3/30/15) FR, 33 (9/25/14) FR, FR 25 (11/1/12)

386-384   Fastest 500 chest-touching-ground pushups in a row (min/sec)   19:13.2 (10/11/15) CR, 21:09.84 (7/4/14) FR, OR 21:34.06 (6/14/14)

383-379 Most pushups on floating paddle board in 4 minutes 129 reps (9/26/15) CR, FR 121 reps (12/20/13), in 2 mins 83 reps (9/26/15) CR, 72 reps (12/20/13) FR, FR 63 rep (12/14/13)

378-375   Most one arm one leg inverted row pull-ups   20 reps (9/24/15) CR, 17 reps (4/1/15) FR, 11 reps (1/8/15) FR, OR 9 reps (9/3/14)

374-372   Most reptile tiger bend pushups in 10 minutes   181 reps (9/21/15) CR, 164 reps (1/8/15) FR, OR 140 reps (10/7/14)

371-369   Most consecutive back-of-hand pushups on a beach   40 reps (9/20/15) CR, 31 (3/30/15) FR, OR 21 (8/23/14)

368-366   Most consecutive under hand false grip inverted row pushups   45 reps (9/20/15) CR, 32 reps (6/12/15) BR, FR 21 reps (1/25/15)

365   Fastest time to do 200 consecutive pushups and 200 meter freestyle swim (min/sec)   OR 7:45.45 (9/6/15)

364-362 Most deep squats and pushups in 2 minutes   166 reps (9/1/15) CR, 161 reps (5/18/15) FR, FR 150 reps (5/14/15)

361-337   Most strict one arm squat thrusts in certain time frames: 5 mins/153 reps (8/31/15) CR, 130 (4/2/15) FR, 115 (1/8/15) FR, 105 (12/31/14) FR, OR 82 (9/1/14), in 4 mins/120 reps (8/31/15) CR, 105 (4/2/15) FR, 95 (1/8/15) FR, 85 (12/31/14) FR, OR 71 (9/1/14), in 3 mins/95 reps (8/31/15) CR, 85 (4/2/15) FR, 76 (1/8/15) FR, 70 (12/31/14) FR, OR 56 (9/1/14), in 2 mins/70 reps (8/31/15) CR, 63 (4/2/15) FR, 57 (1/8/15) FR, 53 (12/31/14) FR, OR 42 (9/1/14) in one min/46 reps (8/31/15) CR, 40 (4/2/15) FR, 36 (1/8/15) FR, 35 (12/31/14) FR, OR 30 (9/1/14)

336-334   Fastest nonstop 40ft L-Sit rope climb   15.52 secs (8/29/15) CR, 15.68 secs (7/18/15) FR, OR 17.83 secs (6/13/15)

333-332   Fastest arms only 20ft rope climb wearing 10-kilogram ankle weights   10.51 secs (8/29/15) CR, OR 12.38 secs (8/2/15)

331-330   Fastest time to do 250 chest-touching-ground tricep pushups   10:17.09 (8/14/15) CR, OR 10:58.9 (8/9/15)

329   Fastest time to do 500 consecutive chest-touching-ground tricep pushups   OR 22:50.6 (8/14/15)

328-321   Most bar dips in one minute 66 reps (8/6/15) CR, 54 reps (6/22/15) FR, 52 reps (1/19/15) FR, 50 reps (7/12/14) FR, 47 reps (11/19/13) BR, 45 reps (5/5/12) FR, OR 43 reps (4/4/12)

320-316   Fastest time to do 100 chin-ups and 100 push-ups 5:00.45 (7/29/15) CR, 6:34.05 (11/23/14) FR, 6:37.39 (10/15/12) FR, 6:48.68 (9/6/12) FR, OR 7:01.3 (7/28/12)

315-313   Most strict chest-touching-ground reptile pushups in one minute 43 reps (7/29/15) CR, 40 reps (9/26/14) FR, OR 21 reps (9/1/14)

312-310   Fastest time to do 100 strict V-Squats with a BOSU (min/sec)   1:46.84 (7/24/15) CR, 1:53 (3/31/15) FR,OR 2:20.53 (12/16/14)

309-308   Fastest nonstop 20ft L-sit rope climb   9.25 secs (7/18/15) CR, OR 10.57 secs (6/13/15)

307-305   Fastest arms only 20ft rope climb   8.24 secs (7/18/15) CR, 8.44 secs (7/11/15) FR, OR 10.16 secs (6/13/15)

304-303   Highest score in leaping mtn. climber and 40 yd archery (max 3 mins)   255 points (7/12/15) CR, OR 204 points (11/6/13)

302   Most 20 archer pull-up and 20 archer push-up cadence test (with 20 sec rest in btw)   OR 2 sets (7/12/15)

301-300   Longest iron cross on parallel bars   39.85 secs (7/4/15) CR, OR 27.5 secs (12/28/14)

299-297 Fastest half-mile cross country run + 10 yd archery bullseye (min/sec) 2:52.3 (6/24/15) CR, 3:19.8 (5/6/14) FR, OR 3:36.7 (10/31/13)

296 Fastest 500 rep bodyweight exercise challenge (any order 100 decline pushups, 100 deep squats with arms held out, 100 bar dips breaking 90 degrees, 100 strict pull-ups and 100 flexed hang knee to elbows)   OR 18:39 min/sec (6/23/15)

295-293 Fastest time to complete 500 chin-ups + 500 push-ups (min/sec) 41:41.62 (6/23/15) CR, 48:53.73 (5/25/12) FR, OR 49:40.65 (3/31/12)

292-291 Longest L-sit hang on the bar (min/sec)   1:29.59 (6/21/15) CR, FR 1:12.12 (4/16/15)

290 Most arms-only rope climb Recordsetter World Records in 30 minutes OR 4 records (6/13/15) *Set for Alicia's parents who are celebrating their 45th anniversary!

289   Fastest nonstop 80ft L-sit rope climb   OR 48.91 seconds (6/13/15)

288-287   Most combined pull-ups and chin-ups in 6 minutes   163 reps (6/6/15) CR, OR 160 reps (1/10/15)

286   Fastest cross country 1600 meter run with 400 deep squats (100 reps per 400m)   OR 13:43.3 (min/sec) (5/30/15)

285-284   Fastest one mile run with 400 chest-touching-ground push-ups (100 reps per 400m)   18:52.08 (5/29/15) CR, OR 22:55 (8/6/12)

283-282   Most consecutive 2-finger strict pull-ups on a straight bar   26 reps (4/28/15) CR, BR 24 reps (2/14/14)

281   Longest pike hold in support on men's gymnastics still rings   CR 64.2 seconds (4/19/15)

280-276   Most consecutive knee tucks with 5lbs ankle weight on both legs   198 reps (4/11/15) CR, 152 reps (11/23/14) FR, 134 reps (12/12/13) FR, 120 reps (6/19/12) FR, OR 103 reps (5/22/12)

275-273 Fastest time to complete 200 elevated leg locked-finger pushups 9:46.85 (4/11/15) CR, 10:33.43 (10/23/13) FR, OR 12:45.43 (6/17/13)

272 — Most one arm 3 finger inverted row pull-ups — OR 15 reps (3/30/15)

271-270 Most consecutive 4 finger egg-on-spoon -in-mouth pullups in a minute — 7 reps (3/28/15) CR, OR 6 reps (5/13/12)

269-267 Most one –arm medicine ball leaping mtn. climber exercise in 5 minutes 520 reps(3/28/15)CR, 376 (12/18/13)FR, OR 308 (11/13/12)

266-265 Most egg-on-spoon-in-mouth L pullups in one minute — 10 reps (3/28/15) CR, OR 8 (6/19/12)

264-262 Most leaping mtn. climber exercises on 2 medicine balls in 5 minutes 558 reps (3/28/15) CR, 538 (12/18/13) FR, OR 440 (11/7/12)

261-260 Most reps in 35 minute strict pull-squat-push challenge (30 mins of pull-ups with 100 deep squats then 5 mins of 10lbs med ball burpee pushups counting reps for the pull-ups and pushups) 503 reps (3/14/15) CR, OR 457 reps (9/20/12)

259-244 Most shoulder-level perfect pullups in time frames: 5 minutes/153 reps (3/12/15) CR, 130 (11/17/14) FR, 121 (8/5/14) FR, 111 (11/16/13) FR, 104 (8/23/13) FR, 102 (7/3/13) FR, OR 99 (6/14/13) in 3 minutes/104 (3/12/15) CR, 90 (11/17/14) FR, 88 (8/5/14) FR, 79 (11/16/13) FR, 71 (8/23/13) FR, 66 (6/14/13) FR, 62 (5/28/13) FR, 54 (5/2/13) FR, OR 52 (3/27/13)

243-242 Most consecutive reptile-pushups in one hour — 858 reps (2/28/15) CR, OR 763 reps (12/12/12)

241-240 Fastest one-leg 500 meter indoor row (rower under 136 lbs) — 2:06.8 (8/23/15) CR, OR 2:09.8 (2/21/15)

239-238 Fastest time to complete 400 rep aerobic capacity wellness challenge 20:23.44 (min/sec) (2/4/15) CR, 23:35.29 (2/4/13) FR, *OR 23:57.69 (2/19/12)

237-236 Most reps of perfect pull-up perfect reptile-pushup challenge in 10 minutes — 160 reps (2/12/15) CR, OR 144 reps (11/12/12)

235-234 Most consecutive quintuple clap pushups — 23 reps (1/25/15) CR, FR 17 reps (4/12/13)

233 — Most consecutive quadruple clap pushups — CR 31 reps (1/25/15)

232-231 Highest Score in towel pull-up pentathlon — 144 reps (1/24/15) CR, OR 122 reps (8/6/12)

230-228 Most consecutive archer pull-ups — 30 reps (1/19/15) CR, 29 reps (7/12/14) FR, OR 28 reps (6/3/14)

227-226 Most consecutive flutter presses with 40% of one's body weight — 155 reps (1/12/15) CR, OR 130 reps (5/17/12)

225-222 Most consecutive strict windshield wiper exercises in minute 55 reps (1/11/15) CR, 50 (9/20/13) FR, 40 (5/1/13) FR, OR 30 (8/16/12)

221-220 Most sports competed in on the elite level with at least one world championship victory 17 sports (1/1/15) CR, OR 16 (4/5/12)

219-218 Most consecutive bar dips with band resistance — 51 dips (12/22/14) CR, FR 41 dips (11/19/13)

217 — Most one-armed Hindu pushups on a basketball — 111 pushups (12/20/14) CR, *FR 30 pushups (2/26/12)

216-215 Longest side-to-side rope pull-ups cadence test (10 per minute till failure) — 30 mins (12/7/14) CR, OR 10 mins (9/8/12)

214-212 Most egg son spoon-in-mouth pullups in minute 17 reps (12/4/14) CR, 16 reps (12/20/12) FR, OR 15 reps (5/13/12)

211-210 Most arms-crossed bent knee sit-ups in 3 minutes — 151 (11/26/14) CR, OR 150 (8/20/14)

209-208 Most reps in 10 minute arms-crossed bent knee situps with knuckle pushups 385 reps (11/26/14) CR, OR 350 reps (1/2/14)

207-196 Most shoulder-level perfect pull-ups in time frames: 30 minutes/568 reps (11/17/14) CR, 514 (8/5/14) FR, 439 (11/16/13) FR, OR 375 (5/4/13), in 15 mins/315 reps (11/17/14) CR, 283 (8/5/14) FR, OR 248 (11/16/13), in 10 mins/223 reps (11/17/14) CR, 206 (8/5/14) FR, OR 186 (11/16/13), in an hour/1,035 reps (11/17/14) CR, OR 822 (11/16/13)

195-194 Most knuckle pushups on a concrete floor in a row 160 reps (10/16/14) CR, 141 reps (8/28/14) BR, *BR 105 reps (2/28/12)

193-191 Longest consecutive cadence strict form spiderman pushups 11 mins (10/12/14) CR, 8 mins (3/11/13) FR, OR 5 mins (5/22/12)

190-189 Longest one-armed plank with feet placed 2ft apart (min/sec) — 9:06.51 (10/7/14) CR, FR 6:36.78 (3/25/12)

188-187 Fastest time to forward crabwalk 100 meters (min/sec) — 1:06.15 (9/10/14) CR, OR 1:41.57 (7/5/12)

186 — Most strict chest-touching-ground reptile-pushups in 5 minutes — OR 72 reps (9/1/14)

185-178 Most one-armed leaping mtn. climber exercise ins 5 minutes/509 reps (8/29/14) CR, 377 (1/22/14) FR, 366 (6/5/13) FR, 342 (11/13/12) FR, 321 (11/2/12) FR, 270 (6/22/12) FR, 226 (6/13/12) BR, OR 130 (3/25/12)

177-171 Most leaping mtn. climber exercise in 5 mins/540 reps (8/29/14) CR, 517 reps (11/8/12) FR, 460 reps (11/13/12) FR, 427 reps (6/22/12) FR, 403 (6/14/12) FR, OR 369 reps (2/26/12)

170 — Fastest time to run Sequoia National Park Sunset Rock Trail 0.7 mile — OR 4:48.58 (8/26/14)

169 — Fastest time to run Sequoia National Park Big Trees Trail 0.6 mile — OR 4:04.50 (8/25/14)

168-167 Fastest 100 meter crabwalk — 54 seconds (8/24/14) CR, OR 57.45 seconds (7/5/12)

166 — Most leaping mtn. climber exercise on a beach in 5 minutes — OR 280 reps (8/23/14)

165 — Most leaping mtn. climber exercise on a beach in one minute — OR 109 reps (8/23/14)

164-162 Most knuckle pushups on a beach in a row 260 reps (8/23/14) CR, 193 reps (6/6/14) FR, FR 105 reps (12/20/13)

161-160 Fastest time to run to Summit of Sugarloaf Mtn. in Clermont, Fl 0.7 mile — 4:58.9 (8/17/14) CR, OR 5:27.92 (5/26/12)

159-158 Fastest time to bicycle to Summit of Sugarloaf Mtn. in Clermont, Fl 0.7 mile — 4:09.87 (8/17/14) CR, OR 4:27.22 (5/26/12)

157-156 Fastest time to do 100 forearm tricep extension pushups and 100 side-to-side V squats 5:07 (8/16/14) CR, OR 7:34.86 (11/25/13)

155-153 Fastest time to complete 100 reptile pushups with 100 jump squats 6:41 (8/16/14) CR, 6:59 (9/6/13) FR, OR 7:42 (5/25/13)

152-151 Fastest triple arm endurance challenge (100 pullups, 100 consecutive reptile pushups, 100 chinups) 17:28.2 (6/12/14) CR, OR 20:37.97 (4/5/13)

Record #	Description	Result/Date
150	Fastest 100 yard beach backward crabwalk	OR 1:18.75 min/sec (6/7/14)
149	Fastest 100 yard beach forward crabwalk	OR 1:52.67 min/sec (6/6/14)
148-147	Highest score in consecutive dips + 40 yard archery obstacle course (max 3 mins)	52 points (5/16/14) CR, OR 49 points (11/4/13)
146-145	Fastest time to perform 100 strict pullups and 10 yd archery bullseye combo	5:58.48 (5/15/14) CR, OR 6:22.8 (10/31/13)
144	Fastest 1500 meter cross country run and 10 yd archery bullseye combo	OR 5:26.35 (5/6/14)
143-142	Fastest 100 deep squat and 10 yd archery bullseye combo	1:55 (5/6/14) CR, OR 2:01.43 (10/31/13)
141-140	Fastest 100 chest-touching-ground pushups and 10 yd archery bullseye combo	3:29.95 (5/6/14) CR, OR 3:58.35 (11/16/13)
139-138	Highest score in inverted row chin-ups with 40 yd archery obstacle course (3 min max)	74 points (5/1/14) CR, OR 65 (1/18/13)
137-136	Highest score in consecutive chin-ups and 40 yd archery obstacle (3 min max)	54 points (5/1/14) CR, OR 53 points (11/11/13)
135-134	Highest score in inverted row pull-ups + 40 yd obstacle archery (3 min max)	68 points (5/1/14) CR, OR 60 points (11/18/13)
133-132	Highest score in consecutive pullups + 40 yd obstacle archery (3 min max)	54 points (5/1/14) CR, OR 50 (10/22/13)
131	Most reps in 20 minute plank calisthenics challenge (5 x min leaping mtn. climber and one min chest-touching-ground pushups) then (5 x minute squat thrusts and min of chest-touching-ground locked finger pushup)	OR 1,136 reps (3/29/14)
130-127	Fastest time to complete 250 consecutive reptile-pushups 12:46.52 (3/20/14) CR, 13:31.56 (8/23/12) FR, 14:16.24 (6/15/12) FR, OR 24:27.29 (5/19/12)	
126-122	Most consecutive side-to-side rope pull-ups	35 (3/11/14) CR, 27 (5/29/13) FR, 25 (2/7/13) FR, 21 (10/9/12) FR, OR 15 (8/26/12)
121	Most consecutive strict one-arm perfect pushups in a 10 minutes (alternating hands)	OR 80 reps (2/4/14)
120-118	Longest TRX 2 medicine ball knee tuck push-up cadence test (15 reps per minute till failure) 5 mins (1/21/14) CR, 4 mins (10/9/12) FR, OR 3 mins (8/29/12)	
117-116	Most reps in 5 mins of leaping mtn. climber variety act (5 different types/min each) 305 reps (1/21/14) CR, OR 298 reps (10/30/12)	
115	Most mtn. climber exercise on knuckles in one minute	CR 260 reps (1/8/14)
114	Most bare knuckle pushups in 15 minutes	OR 326 reps (1/15/14)
113-110	Most arms crossed bent leg situps in 5 minutes/230 reps (1/2/14) CR, 215 reps (5/25/13)FR, 210 reps (2/11/13)FR, OR 190 (1/1/13)	
109-108	Most 10lbs weighted double L challenge (gymnastics floor leg lift, Towel L-pull-up total)	33 reps (12/19/13) CR, OR 21 (12/14/12)
107-106	Most high leaping mtn. climber plyometric alligator pushup challenge reps in 10 mins	168 reps (12/12/13) CR, OR 125 (11/14/12)
105-102	Most consecutive tiger bend pushups with feet on the floor	415 (12/11/13) CR, 260 (1/12/13) FR, 105 (7/29/12) FR, FR 55 (7/11/12)
101-100	Fastest time to complete 100 meter plyometric alligator pushups	9:05 (12/1/13) CR, OR 12:10.75 (11/21/12)
99	Fastest time to complete Clermont Waterfont Park Pier-to-Pier 1k SUP on 12 ft 6 inch board	7:57.15 (11/24/13)
98	Lowest score in 200ft rope climb + 40 yd archery obstacle	OR 6.65 points (11/19/13)
97	Most consecutive plyometric parallel bar dips	CR 35 dips (11/19/13)
96	Highest score in arm walk + 40yd archery obstacle (3 min max)	OR 178 points (11/18/13)
95-94	Highest score in 50ft rope climb + 40 yd archery obstacle	5.58 points (11/6/13) CR, OR 2.27 points (10/22/13)
93-91	Most one leg burpee-pushups in one minute	29 (11/1/13) CR, 26 (11/7/12) BR, OR 21 (8/16/12)
90	Most "archercise" records set on Halloween	OR 4 records (10/31/13)
89	Fastest time for 100 elevated leg lifts + 10 yd archery bullseye combo	OR 4:33.50 (10/31/13)
88-87	Fastest time for 100 consecutive leg lifts on elevation (at least 32 inches at top)	2:50.72 (9/26/13) CR, OR 3:31.70 (5/3/12)
86-84	Longest one-armed dead hang using a towel grip	32.52 seconds (9/20/13) CR, 21.71 secs (8/31/12) FR, FR 16.70 secs (6/19/12)
83-80	Most 180 degree deep squats and 2ft long jumps in 3 minutes	70 reps (9/7/13) CR, 65 (5/8/13) FR, 50 (8/15/12) FR, OR 32 (6/24/12)
79	Longest distance to arm walk on bars in 1 minute	OR 130 ft (7/28/13)
78	Longest distance to arm walk on bars in 5 minutes	OR 340 ft (7/20/13)
77-73	Longest one-armed Chinese Push-up static hold time 7:38 (7/11/13) CR, 6:00 (6/26/13) BR, 2:59 (11/29/13) BR, 1:02.33 (8/11/12) BR, FR 40.48 seconds (6/20/12)	
72	Most consecutive hand waving flexed one-arm hang L-Lifts	OR 8 L-lifts (7/5/13)
71	Longest distance covered in 4 minute variety arm walk challenge	OR 180 ft (7/4/13)
70	Fastest 40ft arm walk in Withlacoochee River Park Tower	OR 1:57 (min/sec) (5/16/13)
69-67	Most situps –flutter crossover reps in 15 minutes	583 reps (4/29/13) CR, 502 reps (8/13/12) FR, OR 472 reps (6/6/12)
66-63	Most consecutive feet together hands at knee straight leg pulses	153 (4/29/13) CR, 80 (4/12/13) BR, 50 (3/29/13) BR, OR 30 (8/13/12)
62	Most burpee box pushups in a minute	CR 33 (2/6/13)
61	Most reps in 13 minute mishmash legathlon (perform 13 leg exercises in a row)	OR 403 reps (2/1/13)
60	Most reps in 13 minute mishmash armathlon (perform 13 arm exercises in a row)	OR 216 reps (1/31/13)
59	Fastest time to perform 100 sand deep squat jumps, while tossing 10lbs medicine ball	OR 5:53 (1/18/13)
58	Most reps in 13 mishmash abathlon (perform 13 ab exercises in a row)	OR 314 reps (1/11/13)

Record #	Description	Result/Date
57	Most reps in 10 minute weighted aerobic strength test	OR 222 reps (1/6/13)
56-55	Fastest 42ft crabwalk	5.7 seconds (12/25/12) CR, FR 6.74 seconds (7/5/12)
54-53	Fastest forward 42ft crabwalk	6.56 seconds (12/25/12) CR, OR 9.08 (7/5/12)
52-51	Fastest 84 feet combo crabwalk (begin 42ft forward, then 42ft backward)	11.53 seconds (12/23/12) CR, OR 12.43 secs (12/17/12)
50	Longest arm walk, while balancing an egg on spoon in mouth	OR 54ft (12/19/12)
49	Highest score in 20 minute exercise "Triple Eggcercise" Challenge	OR 330 points (12/18/12)
48-45	Most alternating squat thrusts in a minute	372 reps (12/15/12) CR, 303 (10/31/12) BR, 232 (10/26/12) BR, BR 206 (10/23/12)
44	Most 10 minute extreme deep squat and pushup variety acts	OR 279 reps (12/11/12)
43	Most bar runner exercises	CR 237 knee lifts (12/10/12)
42	Most triple egg balance BOSU knee tuck and single leg balance perfect pushups	OR 32 reps (12/9/12)
41	Most consecutive knee tuck push-pull challenges	OR 537 reps (12/1/12)
40-39	Most variations of 5 minute leaping mtn. climbers records set in one hour	4 records (11/13/12) CR, OR 3 records (7/30/12)
38	Most opposite one-arm and leg medicine ball leaping mtn. climber exercises in 5 mins	OR 96 reps (11/13/12)
37-36	Most one-legged burpees with opposite one-armed pushups with end jump and clap in minute	12 (11/13/12) CR, OR 10 (8/16/12)
35	Most consecutive chin-ups with 40% of one's body weight held between feet	OR 10 chin-ups (8/26/12)
34	Most consecutive flexed hang knee raise tucks in one minute with 5lbs on each ankle	OR 26 knee lifts (8/26/12)
33	Most windshield wiper exercises in 30 minutes	OR 350 reps (8/24/12)
32	Fastest time to complete 500 consecutive reptile-pushups	OR 32:33.77 (8/23/12)
31	Most reps performed in an abdominal decathlon	OR 1,310 reps (8/13/12)
30	Most chin-ups in 3,30, and 60 minute timed events completed in one bout	CR 3 min/76 reps, 445 reps/30 mins, 760 reps/hour (8/10/12)
29	Most consecutive pull-ups with 40% of one's body weight held between feet	OR 8 reps (8/7/12)
28	Fastest time to complete 1500 meter run and 96 ft arms-only rope climb	OR 7:18.28 (8/3/12)
27	Longest time for 6-12 inch straight leg hold	OR 31:36.58 (8/1/12)
26	Fastest time to complete combo 500 meter run and 36ft arms-only rope climb	OR 2:04.72 (4/31/12)
25	Fastest time to complete 100 meter run and 12ft arms-only rope climb	OR 20.57 seconds (4/31/12)
24-23	Fastest climb in arms-only L-position for 12 feet	3.96 seconds (7/31/12) CR, OR 4.80 seconds (3/9/12)
22	Most opposite arm and leg leaping mtn. climber in 5 minutes	OR 95 reps (7/30/12)
21	Most double bar flexed hang knee tucks in a row with 5lbs on each ankle	OR 48 knee tucks (7/22/12)
20-17	Most push-up/pull-up combos in one minute	20 (7/22/12) CR, 18 (6/9/12) BR, 15 (5/27/12) FR, FR 14 (3/18/12)
16-15	Most sit-ups in 30 minutes with hands held on side of head and elbows touch knees	1,032 sit-ups (7/17/12) CR, OR 927 (4/24/12)
14	Longest cadence back-up exercise (30 reps a minute till failure)	OR 21 minutes (6/24/12)
13	Fastest time in 100 tricep pushups/100 m Freestyle Swim (in 50m pool)	OR 5:41.35 (6/18/12)
12	Most L position ring dips in one minute with 5lbs ankle weights on both legs	OR 5 dips (5/24/12)
11	Longest cadence presses using 40% of one's bodyweight with straight leg hold (25 reps/min till failure)	OR 6 minutes (5/17/12)
10-9	Fastest 400m running medley relay	1:43.12 (5/16/12) CR, OR 1:44.71 (4/28/12)
8	Longest time to hold half-way chin-up L-sit with egg-on-spoon in mouth	OR 1:23.6 min/sec (5/12/12)
7	Most consecutive ring dips with 40% of one's bodyweight held between legs with egg-on-spoon in mouth	OR 4 dips (5/8/12)
6	Most consecutive ring dips in one minute with 40% bodyweight held between feet	OR 10 dips (5/8/12)
5	Longest time to hold one-arm half-way chin-up in L-sit position with egg-on-spoon-in-mouth	OR 11.69 seconds (5/3/12)
4	Most consecutive clapping pushups with feet off the ground	65 (4/17/12) CR, *59 (2/23/12) BR, *BR 54 (2/21/12)
3	Longest time to support body with arms, while extending legs horizontally	OR 1:27.69 (4/5/12)
2	Most Swiss Ball Squats in one minute (must balance on swiss ball and bend knees 90 degrees)	OR 15 (3/29/12)
1	Fastest time to climb arms-only rope in L-sit position wearing 10lbs of weight on ankles on 12 ft	OR 8.95 seconds (3/9/12)
1	Highest non-stop climb on an arms-only rope in one minute (toughest record to set in the 1,000 records!!)	OR 32.46 meters (3/9/12)
1	Most pull-ups on a 10-inch thick bar during a 30 minute 3-in-1 challenge	OR 205 reps (3/6/12)

Additional Records Set in this Time Period, which are Athletic Achievement Records

Record #	Description	Result/Date
1	Fastest time to set 100 total body exercise records upto One Hour Duration	OR 107 days (8/31/12)
2	Fastest time to set 50 exercise records in upper, lower, and core of body	45 days (8/31/12) CR, 62 days (6/24/12)
2	Most exercise records set, running races won, and records of day achieved in a month	39 achievements (8/31/12) CR, OR 35 (5/29/12)
1	Most exercise records set in 7 days in a row (2 records must be at least one hour in duration and all new records)	OR 22 (8/16/12)
1	Most variations of one leg burpee pushup records set in 30 minutes	OR 3 records (8/16/12)
1	Largest variety of ab exercise records set in one hour	OR 4 records (8/13/12)